EASYMEDICINE
HOME-MEDICINE FOR FAMILY-TREATMENT

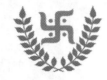

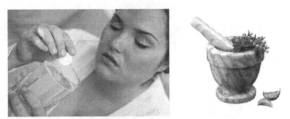

A COMPLETE GUIDE FOR TREATMENT AND MAINTENANCE OF HEALTH

AN USER-FRIENDLY SYSTEM OF TREATMENT FOR CHRONIC AND COMPLEX DISEASES WITH MULTIFARIOUS MEDICINES

AN EASY SOLUTION—SELECT YOUR OWN MEDICINE DISEASE MAY BE MANY, BUT MEDICINES ARE SAME

Author:

DR. BISWAJIT BISWAS
B.Tech (Hons.) IIT Kharagpur, M.B.E.H.

e-mail ID: easymedicine12@gmail.com
                 biopathy1@gmail.com
Website: www.homemedicine.in

A BOOK ON HOME-MEDICINE USEFUL FOR FAMILY AND STUDENTS OF SCIENCE OR NUTRITION

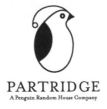

PARTRIDGE
A Penguin Random House Company

To order additional copies of this book, contact
Partridge India
000 800 10062 62
orders.india@partridgepublishing.com

www.partridgepublishing.com/india

CONTENTS

Dedicated to:

THE NATURE, CREATOR OF LIFE

● HERBAL ● HOMEOPATHY ● AYURVEDA ● BIOPATHY ●

PREFACE

The main objective of EASYMEDICINE book is to provide overall knowledge on home-treatment or application of medicine within the family. Most of the time we do not suffer from serious disease. Your child may be suffering from common cold and cough, you may be suffering from gastritis or cardiovascular disease and your parents may be suffering from complex or multiple diseases due to age factor. Often you may not have time and money to even visit doctor.

To overcome the difficulty of treatment of family-members we have selected only 7 or 8 numbers of medicines to simplify the process of treatment. Limited number of medicines means less confusion and application becomes user-friendly. One can get rid of majority of problems with little or no effort by keeping some home-stock of the medicines. Thus the concept of home-treatment is unique in all respect.

This book provides you necessary information on underlying causes of disease and how to treat disease by correcting the disharmony of nervous system, lymphatic system and blood or circulatory system (commonly known as metabolic disorder). Disturbance of these three systems is mainly responsible for disease. Hence it is better to treat only the "metabolic disorder" instead of applying medicine for each type of disease. This concept is widely applied for treatment of complex diseases under home-treatment or family-treatment. In case of sudden onset of disease apply your home-stock medicine first at "zero-hour" to simplify the case—then take your own decision.

Diet and exercise also play vital role for maintenance of health. Unfortunately we do not pay much attention on appropriate diet and physical exercise. Additionally, majority of us are directly or indirectly affected by high-order environmental pollution, resulting from water-pollution, air-pollution, food-pollution and microwave-pollution. Considering all these limitations a simplified schema or plan of maintenance of health is highlighted in this book— with an objective of preventing the dreadful diseases. We especially focus on "Preventive Medicine" which one should follow to avoid complicated diseases. Remember the old proverb—"Prevention is better than cure".

Another advantage of home-treatment is that there is no "fixed rule" or "dose" of taking medicine. All medicines are non-toxic and absolutely free from side effects. Therefore you need not worry about "dose" of the medicine. One can take the medicines in most flexible way.

It should be however remembered that treatment of Surgery, Emergency and High-order Genetic Diseases must be done under allopathic system of medicine by Specialist Doctors. One must be well aware with limitations of the system of home-treatment.

The book "EASYMEDICINE" is written on the background of the desire of our patients who frequently seek detail and logical explanation on the method of family-treatment—thus benefiting them as well as others. By keeping this book at home one will get acquainted with the philosophy of home-treatment and application of the medicines.

One must however note that the most important aspect for maintenance of health, even treatment of so-called complex diseases, is extensive use of "*Natural Medicines*". These "natural medicines" are Chlorophyll and Coloured Pigments (Bioflavonoid), available plenty in Nature from fresh fruits, vegetables, green leaves and non-toxic coloured flowers. As a matter of fact treatment by using our "medicines" is of least importance—medicines referred in the book are actually meant for the people who are not familiar with the "*amazing curative power of natural medicines*". I have therefore repeatedly emphasized the importance of "*bio-force*" or "*bio-energy*" in my book. It is needless to say that purest form of "*bio-force*" is only available in chlorophyll and coloured pigments of *Nature*. Read the "basic causes of disease" and "genetic relationship between disease and longevity" mentioned at Chapters-1 & 3—you will be certainly able to find out the *easy-solution* for maintenance of health as well as treatment of diseases!

I hereby take the opportunity to acknowledge deep gratitude to my daughter Dr. Srijita Biswas and my students Dr. Soma Ghosh and Sailaja Vanapalli for their enthusiasm and co-operation in the preparation of the manuscript. I express my heartiest gratitude to my colleague Dr. Tapan Biswas, MBBS, DGO, for thorough checking of the book especially with respect to present-day nutritional concept. For overall supervision, I owe not a little to my friend Dr. Saurabh Kumar.

Finally, I remain very much thankful to M/s PARTRIDGE, for undertaking the responsibility of publishing this book.

Hope students belonging to science or nutrition group will find this book logical and interesting in all respect.

Dr. Biswajit Biswas
(Mob.: +919433931994)

Block-EB, Plot-64, 1848 Rajdanga Main Road
Kolkata-700107, India
Date: 15 April 2014

Chapter-1: General

Introduction to Home-Medicine

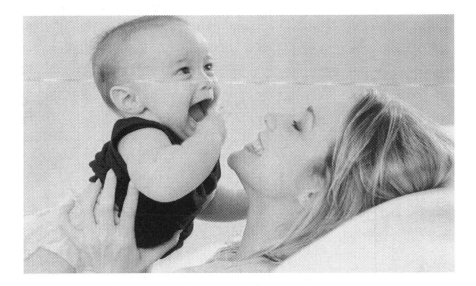

Before we peer into the modern age today, we were purely dependent on the nature for treatment. Medicinal plant and trees, herbs and creepers, soil and mineral sources, etc. were used abundantly in treatment of diseases. Our olden "Ayurveda Shastra" and medicinal treatment are the glaring example of above. On the pace of civilization, people are getting off from ayurveda and herbal medicines, soil, mineral resources, etc. and precarious diseases of complex types are being influenced rapidly. Besides there are various types of problem such as environmental pollution, extensive use of chemical manures and pesticides in agriculture, taking of adulterated and preservative-added food and microwave pollution. We cannot forsake modern civilization—so to solve the problems principally depending upon natural resources, we have introduced necessary medicines for home-treatment to cure disease in easy process. The characteristic of treatment is fundamental in all respect as mentioned below:

- All medicines are made of non-toxic materials of Ayurvedic (Indian Science of Medicine), Herbal and Biochemic ingredients. The non-toxic medicines are all free from reaction and there is no particular direction for use. So no dose is earmarked for use the medicines—because there is no harm if taken in excess. The medicines are user-friendly and can be selected or applied easily.

- The medicines for patient are prepared by our own specialist doctors—for our aim is to raise the quality of medicines and for the welfare of people, we do not keep profit on medicines. As a result the medicines are not being made commercially and not sold through any shop. The medicines are to be directly taken by the patient from us for their own use. Besides to raise multifarious character of the medicines, the ingredients of medicines are upgraded from time to time for the need of improvement.

- Each and every medicine can be used in various diseases—even herbal medicines if taken along with the system of medicines of allopathy and homeopathy, give better benefit.

- No particular time is earmarked for taking medicines—the medicines can be taken at any time at one's own will in a day. No restriction of food is related to taking of medicines—sour, bitter, hot and sweet, any type of food can be taken. But keeping $1/3^{rd}$ of the stomach empty, light food is scientific.

- Everyday some green leaves and coloured vegetables and fruits in the form of juice or salad in un-cooked or raw condition should be taken. As a result, efficiency of every cell of in the body increases. On practice of the above food habit during treatment, you are sure to get better result.

- If the medicines are taken for long in healthy condition, it ensures longer life.

- The main objective of our medicines and our treatment is to keep set right function of digestion and nerves—so that keeping away metabolic disorder, the body will earn health. To remain disease-free, we recommend the use of BIO-TONE PLUS, BOOSTER, BIO-HERB, SUGAR-TABLET or LIV-TREAT, SHAKTI-RAJ and DANTA-RAJ for the entire life. Besides if eye sight is not all right, mental peace gets disturbed, so we advice to use non-irritant type HERBAL EYE-DROP. If digestion and eye care continued in proper way, the pleasure of body and mind keeps intact. So all the above medicines are counted as "Basic Medicines" for "metabolic disorder" and should be continued for the whole life. These are applicable to all—youngsters as well as old.

- It is a well known fact that disease is caused due to disharmony of nervous system, lymphatic system and blood or circulatory system. All the three systems are interdependent to each other—disturbance of one will affect the other. Hence it is very difficult to pinpoint the exact cause of disease, especially when the disease is of chronic, multiple and complex type. The easiest solution is therefore, to treat the metabolic disorder only by applying few medicines, instead of applying array of medicines for each type of disease. The treatment is thus simplified by improving overall health or condition of the patient.

The book EASYMEDICINE gives preliminary guidance or information on treatment of chronic and complex diseases. Medicines are widely used as "Preventive" as well as "Curative" in the process of treatment and maintenance of health.

It should be however, noted that no guidance has been highlighted for treatment of Surgery, Emergency and High-order Genetic Diseases, for which treatment under allopathic medicine by Specialist Doctors is compulsory.

* * *

LIST OF DISEASES WHERE MEDICINES ARE APPLICABLE

- Diseases of Infants and Children—Fever, Cold, Cough, Stomach Problem, Tonsillitis, Bronchitis, Throat Pain, Asthma, Food Allergy, Dust Allergy, Skin Disease, etc. Health tonic for growing children.

- Chronic Skin Disease, Itching, Eczema, Psoriasis, Arsenic Poisoning.

- Neurological Diseases—Acute Vertigo, Migraine, Parkinson's Disease, Epilepsy, Flashing sensation of Nerves, Erratic and Shooting Pain, Debility of Nerves, etc.

- Diabetes Mellitus (i.e. Type-2) or Blood Sugar, Diabetic Neuropathy.

- Acidity, gastritis, weakness of digestion, Bleeding Piles, Fistula, Constipation.

- Allergy of all types—Dust Allergy, Food Allergy.

- High Pressure, High Cholesterol and Cardiovascular Diseases.

- Hypothyroidism, Hyperthyroidism, Disease of Glands.

- Disease of Respiratory System—Chronic Cold and Cough, Bronchitis, Pneumonia, Asthma.

- Cancer, Breast and Uterine Tumour—Treatment and prevention.

- Arthritis, Gout, Joint Pain, Nerve and Muscle Pain, Sciatica, Frozen Shoulder, Tennis Elbow.

- Disease of Gum, Mouth and Teeth—Pyorrhea, Spongy Gum, Bleeding and Swelling of Gum, Foul Breath, Ulcer on Tongue and Mouth, etc.

- General and Special Eye Diseases e.g. Glaucoma. Giving-up Spectacles of Children and Youngsters having moderate Power.

- Psychiatry diseases for non-violent and co-operative type patients willing to take our medicines.

• Female Diseases e.g. Leucorrhoea, Menstrual Pain, Excessive Bleeding, etc. Health tonic for pregnant mothers.	• Old Age Problems— Geriatric Diseases e.g. Weakness of Nerves and Digestive System, Shortfall of Memory, Bronchial Problems, etc.
• Disease of Liver—Fatty Liver Disease, Jaundice, Enlargement of Liver.	• General Maintenance of Health—To avoid Surgery and Dreadful Diseases in life, to increase longevity.

NOTE:

1) No medicine for surgery, emergency treatment and high-order genetic diseases is available.

2) Serious and difficult cases must be treated under allopathic system of medicine by specialist doctors.

* * *

RULE FOR USE OF BASIC MEDICINE AND DOSAGE ABOUT

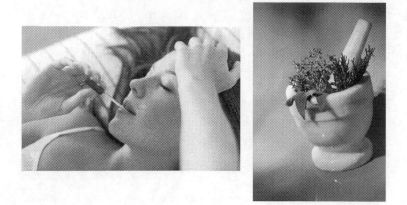

As all our medicines are prepared of non-toxic ingredients, no side effect is caused and no dosage is directed. The word "Dose" is used in toxic group of drugs i.e. if crosses the limit of taking medicine it will make more harm than benefit. Our foods—rice, bread, pulse, grams and nuts, vegetables and fruits are all non-toxic, so we maintain no limit of taking foods i.e. no dose or limit is observed; we can take as much food as we like and any time. Our medicines are also like food or nutrient, if taken in large quantity no side effect comes to spell our body and so the word "Dose" is meaningless to us—medicines can be taken at any time in any quantity we like. Still for general convenience we are trying to give an idea as follows for use of seven basic medicines for "metabolic disorder".

1) BIO-TONE PLUS—It is better to take 1 dose daily for normal maintenance of health. However, depending on the severity of disease, the medicine is to be repeated twice, thrice or even four times in a day. Medicine can be taken in empty stomach as well as in full stomach and there is no restriction of food (sour, sweet, bitter and so on) whatsoever. Apply the medicine in all diseases e.g. fever, cold and cough, arthritis, fatty liver disease, cardiovascular disease, psoriasis, thyroid,

diabetes or even cancer. Medicine acts on nervous system, glands, bones, muscles and all internal organs of the body.

2) BOOSTER—It is better to take 1 dose daily (or half or one-third quantity of Bio-Tone Plus) for normal maintenance of health. Medicine should be preferably taken in combination or alteration of Bio-Tone Plus. Action of this medicine is almost similar to Bio-Tone Plus and should be repeated to twice, thrice or four times daily, depending on severity of disease.

It is to be remembered that Bio-Tone Plus and Booster are complimentary to each other—best result is observed if these two medicines are taken in combination generally in 2:1 or 3:1 ratio. You need not alternate the medicines frequently—start taking high doses of both the medicines daily for 2-3 weeks, thereafter consume one packet of one variety after another without alteration of the same daily. For example, take 2 packets Bio-Tone and 1 packet Booster in a month or 3 packets Bio-Tone and 1 packet Booster in a month. Consume your monthly quota of the medicine in most flexible or random way as per your convenience without making specific schedule or routine of taking medicine daily. However, for your own convenience fix up some dose and time for taking these powder medicines—say 1 or 2 doses of Bio-Tone Plus for 20 days and 1 dose Booster for 10 days to be taken in the morning or in the evening or night. Alternatively, you can also take both the medicines at the same time (say in the morning or evening) instead of taking in two different times of the day.

3) SUGAR-TABLET OR LIV-TREAT—It is better to take 5-6 tablets immediately after taking food. Tablets are bitter, swallow it with water. If taken regularly it purifies 'bile', alters pH of the food to less acidic (note that the stomach fluid is highly acidic in nature, pH varying from 1 to 3). Besides it helps to remove chronic dysentery or amebiasis. Everybody knows almost 80% of people in tropical and coastal region suffer from amebiasis, which is the main cause of constipation. Take anyone of these two medicines to eradicate the problem.

4) SHAKTI-RAJ—It is better to take 2-3 caps of medicine once or twice daily immediately after lunch or dinner or breakfast. Medicine can be taken by the people of all ages—child, adult and old. It is the specific remedy for glaucoma patients. If felt excessively sour, add some water in it.

5) BIO-HERBs—It is better to take 3-4 spoons medicine before going to bed or in the morning in empty stomach. Plenty of water is to be taken along with the medicine. Take some powder of medicine and water in mouth, gurgle and swallow. Dietary fibers will expel toxins from the body through soft stool and will remove flatulence, gas and acidity, loss of appetite and other digestive problems in the long run.

6) DANTA-RAJ—Brush teeth twice daily in the morning and at night with herbal toothpowder. It will also supplement the demand of magnesium of body everyday. It does not diminish the secretion of saliva as it has no foam-creating chemical in it. Everybody knows reduction of secretion of saliva creates various types of disease as saliva is indispensable for digestion.

7) HERBAL EYE-DROP—Apply once at night one or two drops on each eye. Those who are exposed to microwave pollution or dust pollution or watch T.V. or work on computer, apply at least twice daily (no harm if more)—in the morning and at night. The eye-drop is of non-irritant type, is painless and removes eye stress. It comforts eyes and indirectly helps to remove brain excitement and depression and possibilities of cataract in future. Herbal eye-drop however can be replaced by diluting Multi-Care or Aqua-Fresh lotion in a glass or cup of water and then applying on eyes (refer Table-X).

All these seven types of medicines are used as "Basic platform of home-treatment".

HOW LONG THE MEDICINES ARE TO BE USED

The above medicines are invaluable to remove "metabolic disorder" of the body. It is better to use the medicines for whole life—because toxins always get in the body from outside and also created by the body separately. This toxin or poison comes out of body through kidney (urethra), rectum (anus), lung (nose) and skin (sweat glands). Especially because after 30-35 years of age the capabilities of these organs start decreasing, excess toxins accumulates in the body. The above medicines help maintain capabilities of various organs and remove the excess toxin. As a result it reduces the possibilities of getting complicated diseases like diabetes, cardiovascular disease, gall stone, appendicitis, cancer, AIDS, etc. and helps give longer life.

* * *

FIVE "CARES" FOR HEALTH CAN KEEP DISEASE AWAY

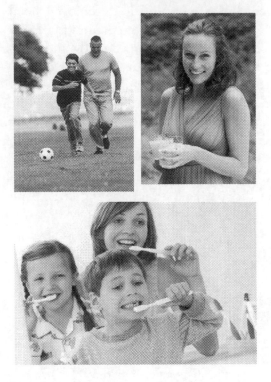

Do you know a little awareness on health can keep you free from serious and complicated diseases like arthritis, diabetes, cardiovascular disease, respiratory disease, gastrointestinal disease, food and dust allergy, neurological and mental disorders, cancer and even AIDS? In modern age our lifestyle and pattern of job has become so complicated and dynamic that teachers, engineers, businessmen, computer professionals, etc. can hardly afford to lead disciplined life till their retirement. In fact it is useless to advice them to do exercise, select pesticide-free and preservative-free foods and to perform Yoga and meditation honestly. It is also useless to advice the urban people to live in countryside to avoid dust, smoke and air pollution, and to breathe oxygen-enriched air. It is not possible to avoid fluoride poisoning and arsenic poisoning resulting from the water we use everyday. Likewise, it is fruitless to advice smokers to give up the habit of smoking which he has started for many years.

A little thought will make you realize that majority of people are unable to maintain their health through appropriate diet and systematic Yoga, meditation and exercise. Moreover, you need special trainer or teacher and environment from which you might get proper guidance and enthusiasm. Due to scarcity of time in modern times, one will perhaps realize that majority of young people cannot afford to follow this "tough and disciplined path" for maintenance of health.

What is then the solution of health maintenance for the urban population, especially the working people and professionals? Modern civilization, modern lifestyle, complex and complicated society, unit-family and environment have gifted us array of complicated or complex diseases. Time has come when we should think for an alternate and easy solution without blaming the victims of the disease. Simple attention or care can make your body free from disease.

Another point need to be mentioned—disease is generally noticed from the middle age, but the underlying cause of disease is the negligence on health in the childhood, the golden period of life. Therefore, one must put special attention on maintenance of health from the childhood or adult so that they do not become victim of complex diseases at their middle age.

LEARN THE FIVE "CARES"

Mouth and Tooth Care:

Starting point of the digestive system is mouth and teeth. Pay special attention on "oral hygiene", which is responsible for majority of stomach troubles. Brush your teeth with 'Danta-Raj' herbal toothpowder twice daily (i.e. morning and evening) using hard brush.

The powder will not only ensure you bacteria-free mouth, but also prevents fluoride-contamination and supplement magnesium to keep your nervous system healthy.

Apply few drops 'Multi-Care' herbal lotion on your gum and massage, at least twice or thrice in a week to keep the gum healthy and hard. Swallow the lotion after massage.

Stomach Care, Purification of Blood:

For better assimilation of food and nutrients, take 6-8 tablets Sugar-Tablet or Liv-Treat, 2-3 caps Shakti-Raj and 3-4 spoons Bio-Herb daily. Sugar-Tablet or Liv-Treat corrects pH value of the food consumed (by neutralizing excess acid of the food), while Shakti-Raj controls blood cholesterol and Bio-Herbs expel toxins and provide 'natural vitamins' and 'dietary fiber'.

Take 1-2 packets Bio-Tone Plus and 1 packet Booster in a month to keep nerves and glands active. These two medicines will also help to protect your lung from air-pollution, smoke and dust. Remember, lung is the important organ for purification of blood, where oxygen enters into blood and carbon dioxide is removed from blood.

It is worth mentioning here that you should never eat full-stomach— always keep your stomach half or one-third empty.

Cleaning of Intestine and Waste Product:

Rectum and kidney play vital role in detoxification of the body. Constipation is the result of improper dietary habit and weakness of rectum nerves. To avoid constipation in general, take plenty of Bio-Herb No. 1 or 2 everyday, say 3-4 spoons either before going to bed or in the morning. Take plenty of water in the morning in empty stomach.

Additionally take Bio-Tone Plus, Booster, Sugar-Tablet or Liv-Treat and Shakti-Raj to improve the function of internal organs.

Skin Care:

Aqua-Fresh herbal bath ensures nourishment of skin, removes harmful bacteria and micro-organisms. It also removes micro-particles of soap used during bath, thus keeps the skin soft and smooth. Medicine cleans sweat-glands of the skin. It is high grade cosmetic and skin-care lotion for ladies and especially infants and children.

Along with it oral medicines are Bio-Tone Plus, Booster, Bio-Herbs, Sugar-Tablet or Liv-Treat and Shakti-Raj—if taken regularly, glossiness of skin increases.

Eye Care:

Eye is an important organ of the head, connected with millions of sensitive nerves. Healthy eyesight increases cheerfulness of mind. To protect the eye from external pollution, dust and microwave pollution, apply herbal eye-drop at least once before going to bed. Eye-drop will remove stress of your eyes and you will feel comfortable before going to sleep.

Children having moderate power of eyes can easily give up spectacles by taking Bio-Tone Plus, Booster, Shakti-Raj and using Danta-Raj and Eye-Drop on long term basis.

IMPORTANT TO NOTE

Bio-Tone Plus and Booster should be taken regularly to keep harmony between the three fundamental systems of the body—nerve, lymph and blood. These two medicines efficiently protect lung from any type of air pollution—its profound action on cleansing process of the lung indicate compulsory application for the urban people, aged, very old and especially smokers.

Sugar-Tablet or Liv-Treat (6-8 tablets) and Shakti-Raj (1-2 caps) should be taken together at least once daily with food for better assimilation of nutrients from food. These two remedies will eradicate cancerous tendency, if taken for whole life.

Bio-Herbs will provide necessary 'natural vitamins' and 'dietary fiber' to detoxify harmful pesticides and preservatives consumed by us everyday along with the food.

*　　*　　*

CHILDREN'S HEALTH CARE AND GUIDE FOR TREATMENT—INFANTS AND BABIES

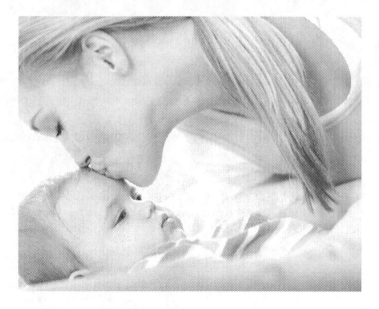

Our medicines are very much effective and helpful for application on infants and babies. Up to 6 months of age, infants should be fed only mother's milk (i.e. breast feeding) to develop immunity. During this period it is important that lactating mother should take the health tonic themselves, a process through which the immunity of mother gets transferred to their child.

Lactating mothers should take 1 or 2 doses Bio-Tone Plus and 1 dose Booster daily, which will not only keep the mother away from disease, but also will help indirectly the infants to develop their immunity to fight against disease.

In addition to above, mothers should take General medicines (Sugar-Tablet or Liv-Treat, Shakti-Raj, Bio-Herb, Danta-Raj and Herbal Eye-Drop) to cover overall maintenance of health.

To keep the skin of the infants and babies bacteria-free, mix 3-4 droppers 'Aqua-Fresh' dilute herbal lotion or few drops 'Multi-Care' concentrate herbal lotion in Olive Oil and apply on the body. These herbal lotions are excellent for protection of skin from bacterial and fungal infections.

Treatment of infants simplified:

Most of the times, babies fall sick due to fever, cold, cough and stomach disorder. Bio-Tone Plus, Booster, Fever-Cold and Stomach-Stool are sufficient to cover all these problems. If the infants are not habituated with solid food or depend only on mother's milk, the medicines are to be taken by mother so that babies receive a small part of medicine through mother's milk. However, most of the cases babies do not feel discomfort if few drops of liquid medicines 'Fever-Cold' or 'Stomach-Stool' is given on baby's tongue or fed by mixing with water or milk. All these medicines are very effective to cure the ailments of babies.

GROWN-UP CHILDREN

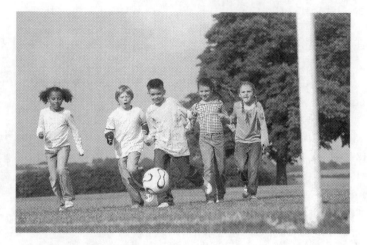

<u>Fever, Cold, Tonsillitis, Dust Allergy, etc:</u>

Apply 'Bio-Tone Plus' and 'Booster' confidently in all cases such as fever, cold, cough, influenza, swelling of tonsil and glands, throat pain, etc. Depending on the severity of the disease, repeat both the medicines several times on the very first day, which may be reduced subsequently on the following days.

Children susceptible to cold and cough, dust allergy, etc. should be given these medicines for the whole year.

<u>Constipation, Diarrhea, Gas, etc:</u>

Main medicine is 'Stomach-Stool'. Besides it is better to take Bio-Tone Plus and Booster regularly on long term basis to improve digestive power and to eradicate constipation.

In case of severe diarrhea and vomiting, mix 4-5 full droppers Multi-Care herbal antibacterial lotion with 6-8 caps Shakti-Raj in a glass of water. Take frequent doses of above mixture and finish the medicine within half an hour. You will be astonished to observe the result. Alternatively, take repeated doses of Stomach-Stool; say at 10-15 minutes interval, till the problem subsides.

Increase of memory and talent:

Ideal medicines are Bio-Tone Plus, Booster and Shakti-Raj. If taken by students of school and college regularly, attention and memory increases and better result in examination is expected.

Additionally, Sugar-Tablet or Liv-Treat should be taken to improve Liver function, eradication of worms, chronic dysentery and purification of blood.

Mouth and Tooth Care:

To make up deficiency of magnesium, make habit of your children to use fluoride-free Danta-Raj herbal toothpowder for brushing teeth twice daily.

Skin Care:

Aqua-Fresh is an ideal cosmetic as well as good antiseptic and antifungal lotion for skin care. It is especially suitable for infants and babies. Besides, use Sugar-Tablet or Liv-Treat and Shakti-Raj regularly. Additionally Bio-Tone Plus and Booster are very much useful in any type of skin disease, as well as to restore glamour of the skin.

Eye Care and diseases:

To avoid influence of pollution of air, computer and T.V., use special herbal eye-drop. Besides to keep good eyesight and to arrest power of the spectacles, take Bio-Tone Plus, Booster and Shakti-Raj regularly.

Do you know majority of children having moderate power of eye can easily give up spectacles? Take Bio-Tone Plus and Booster on long term basis and check the power periodically. These two medicines are wonderful to restore eyesight as well as general health of children.

* * *

HEALTH CARE FOR PREGNANT AND LACTATING MOTHERS

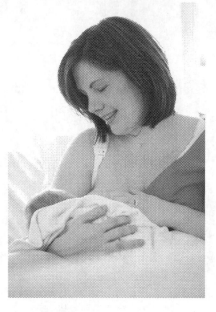

Prime importance should be given on health care of the pregnant mothers to eradicate many complications at the time of delivery and post-natal complications.

Pregnant mothers should take 1-2 doses Bio-Tone Plus and 1 dose Booster daily during their whole term of pregnancy or at least for the last 4-5 months. This will not only help the basic systems (nerve, lymph and blood) of their body to function in a better way, but also will help to develop immunity system of the child after birth. In addition to above, chance of transfer of low-grade genetic diseases from the mother to child reduces to a great extent.

Additionally take General medicines (Sugar-Tablet or Liv-Treat, Shakti-Raj, Bio-Herb) and use Danta-Raj and Eye-Drop for overall maintenance of health during pregnancy.

Take green chlorophyll and coloured pigments (bioflavonoid) in the form of salad or 2-3 glasses fresh fruit juice to be taken in empty stomach in the morning daily, instead of taking artificial vitamins.

Conduct ultrasonography (USG) once under the guidance of a Gynecologist or Radiologist to check the status of the womb.

After the childbirth, continue all above health-tonics at least upto the lactating period to ensure better development of health, immunity system and memory of your child.

*   *   *

FIRSTLY MAKE BACTERIA-FREE MOUTH AND TEETH

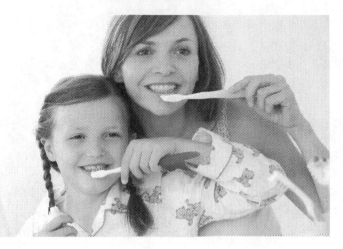

Main principle of health care is bacteria-free mouth and teeth. If care is taken for mouth and teeth, harmful bacteria cannot make entry in stomach—as a result many diseases can be prevented, especially the stomach diseases. If you take rotten food—you will suffer from stomach disorder, similarly if you do not make your mouth bacteria-free, you will surely suffer from various types of stomach problem such as acidity and gas, weakness of digestion and so on. In fact half of the stomach problems are directly related to careless maintenance of mouth and teeth.

Besides, the underlying cause of general metabolic disorders such as arthritis, diabetes, high blood pressure, high cholesterol, heart disease, etc., are related to faulty assimilation of food and nutrients, which is again closely related to weakness of the digestive system.

Therefore, to start with treatment for any chronic disease, it is mandatory to make your mouth bacteria-free by cleaning your teeth by Danta-Raj herbal toothpowder, which is also fluoride-free toothpowder and supplements magnesium in your body.

> *Easiest way to prevent all Stomach problems as well as Dental problems—is to keep your Mouth and Gum bacteria-free and healthy.*

AVOID FLUORIDE POISONING

Use *DANTA-RAJ* Herbal Toothpowder twice daily at morning and night with brush application.

Apply few drops *MULTI-CARE* Herbal Lotion on your gum and massage for few minutes and then swallow the medicine (lotion will also reduce your stomach problem). Apply at least twice or thrice in a week.

Useful tips for removing black spots of smokers:

Take baking powder (used for preparation of cake, pastry, etc.) of good quality and rub your teeth by applying pressure. Clean your mouth by water. Repeat this for few times. By this process black spots of the teeth (nicotine spots or grayish colour of teeth due to tobacco-smoking or excessive iron in water) will be removed very easily. Never use muriatic acid or similar type of lotion—the enamel of teeth will get eroded!

*   *   *

WHY DETOXIFICATION IS NECESSARY FOR TREATMENT OF ALL CHRONIC DISEASES?

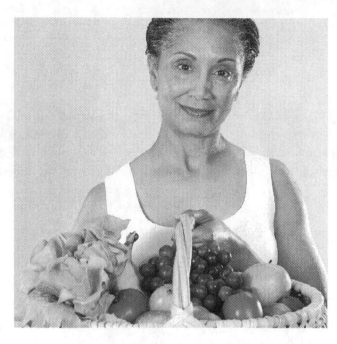

Detoxification is a new concept recently introduced in medical science. Considerable amount of toxin is accumulated in our body which causes illness or disease. Toxin causes micro-inflammation or irritation in body cells and therefore it is essential to remove toxin from the body—thus eliminating the root cause of disease. How toxins are accumulated in our body? The answer is i) from external sources and ii) self-generated source.

TOXINS ACCUMULATED FROM EXTERNAL SOURCES:

Food and agriculture:

Lethal dose of toxins is accumulated in the body everyday from our daily food. Harmful chemicals and poisonous pesticides are extensively used in modern agriculture. Moreover, chemicals are used as preservatives for most of the vegetables, packed foods, sweets and almost all types of junk-foods. Use of artificial manures and genetically modified foods and vegetables are also major source of pollution. As a result, we find increase of diseases of digestive system, diabetes, cardiovascular disease, cancer and especially neurological diseases.

Drinking water:

Due to continuous use of ground water for irrigation, we are facing problems of Fluoride poisoning and Arsenic poisoning. Fluorine is the most reactive element known and readily attacks calcium of bone, which causes arthritis. It also reacts with positive ions (Mg, Fe, etc.) of the body causing disturbance of enzyme function. Similarly, skin disease is spreading because of Arsenic poisoning. Another threat of contamination of drinking water is from industrial waste, which ultimately mixes with drinking water. People residing in industrial belts become victim of industrial waste (from chemical factory) through water, which is sometimes found to be totally unsafe for use.

Air Pollution:

People residing in urban areas and industrial belts are subjected to air pollution through dust, carbon monoxide, lead poisoning and especially heavy metal pollution near steel factories. These are the root cause of respiratory problems of various types e.g. chronic cough, bronchitis, asthma, pneumonia, lung cancer and so on. Increase of lung cancer is mainly due to heavy-metal industrial pollution in air, which is perhaps more serious than tobacco smoking.

Microwave and electromagnetic pollution:

It is comparatively a recent problem developed due to extensive use of T.V., computers, domestic appliances such as micro-oven, mobile phones and especially the transmitting towers. The problem of microwave pollution is largely found in urban areas however, rural areas are not free from the pollution. Young generation who extensively use computers, T.V., mobile phones are the major sufferers of neurological problems such as attention disorder, eye disease, hearing deficiency and even impotency.

It is evident that modern civilization cannot avoid threat of pollution-based toxins derived from food and agricultural pollution, drinking water pollution, air pollution and above all microwave and electromagnetic pollution. On the other hand, do you know that harmful toxins are equally generated by our body itself?

SELF-GENERATED TOXINS:

Toxins from Metabolic Disorders:

During the process of metabolism, a certain portion of food is converted into chemical energy. The unused material is excreted from the body in the form of stool, urine, carbon dioxide, ammonia and sweat. The role of excretory process or mechanism is very important in our body function. Lung, rectum, kidney and skin are the major organs to expel the waste of our body. If the function of any of these organs is affected by some reason, the waste accumulates in our body, which behaves like toxin. Diabetic patients developing high level of urea creatinine is a typical example of self-generated toxin. Therefore, any imbalance or deficiency of function of the system can generate large amount of toxin in our body, which is termed as "metabolic disorder".

Toxins from Pathogenic origin:

Acute or sudden type disease caused by bacteria, parasites and virus is an example of self-generated toxin. Similarly, the reason for fever is due to high rise of toxin in our body, caused by the attack of micro-organisms. Many people will argue that toxins are brought externally by these micro-organisms, but this is not true. Malarial parasites can exist in both mosquito and human being, but human body is attacked with malaria whereas mosquito is not attacked by the disease. In fact the toxin is generated by the defensive or immunity mechanism of the body (B and T lymphocytes, Plasma cells, Macrophages and Dendritic cells) coming in contact with harmful organism (antigen).

DETOXIFICATION—HOW TO EXPEL TOXINS?

Importance of detoxification is overlooked in most of the cases. Hence, treatment of diseases remains incomplete, especially for the treatment of chronic or long lasting diseases.

We provide special attention on detoxification in our system of treatment. Toxins are the root cause of all diseases. It silently produces local or general inflammation (irritation) of cells in our body in varying magnitude. Function of internal organs and glands, lymph, blood, nerves, etc. are greatly affected by the "endurance limit" of the body to withstand accumulated toxins from external sources as well as self-generated source. When the accumulation of toxin crosses threshold level, the body starts to react. This condition is termed as "disease", it may be simple type fever, arthritis, diabetes, cardiovascular disease, cancer, neurological problems and so on.

Keeping this in mind, we have developed medicine to expel the toxins in two ways: i) Direct way and ii) Indirect way.

Direct way of Detoxification:

Bio-Herb Nos. 1 & 2 are the medicines for detoxification in direct way or by rapid method. These are essential medicines used for treatment of all chronic diseases. Medicines are rich with dietary fiber, natural vitamins and Biochemic medicines and are essential to accelerate the process of cure. By intake of these medicines regularly, toxins will be expelled from body in shortest time through stool. For example, people suffering from gout resulting from deposition of uric acid crystal, will feel comfortable within 5 or 6 hours after passing soft or liquid stool, if large amount of Bio-Herb is taken, whereas no other medicine can provide such rapid relief or cure without any side effect. If taken regularly, one need not be worried about detoxification or the process of expelling toxins from body.

Indirect way of Detoxification:

Bio-Tone Plus and Booster are the medicines for improving function of nerves, glands and vital organs of the body such as lung, liver, heart and kidney. If these medicines are taken regularly, function of the vital organs increases and assist to expel the toxins from the body. This process is called indirect method of detoxification. Though the process is slow, medicines are highly effective and useful for treatment of all diseases, irrespective of age and sex whatsoever.

It should be remembered that without a clear concept of detoxification, treatment of chronic disease remains incomplete. Follow the theory of detoxification; you will get wonderful result during treatment of so-called incurable diseases such as arthritis, gout, cardiovascular disease, diabetes, cancer and all types of skin disease, even psoriasis.

*   *   *

LACK OF DIETARY FIBER IS ROOT-CAUSE OF DISEASE

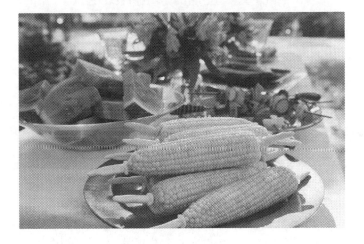

Do you know fiber plays the most important role in maintenance of our health? It is difficult to believe that fiber grows immunity potential of the body to a large extent, whereas contrary to our conventional belief, artificial vitamins play no significant role to develop immunity. On the other hand, our body is capable of developing large number of vitamins. We also get vitamins from our daily food. It has been now established that there is practically no need of taking artificial vitamins—in fact regular intake of artificial vitamins and antioxidants is harmful for health and even reduces longevity. We will be benefited if we concentrate our thoughts on dietary fiber, rather than vitamins.

Our herbal medicines (mixed with Biochemic medicines) Bio-Herb Nos. 1 & 2 are highly efficient to expel toxins accumulated by the food-processing system (i.e. digestive and excretory organs) of the body. Scientists are now convinced with the importance of dietary fiber, because fibers can expel toxins in most efficient way. If you think a little deeper, you will be surprised to learn that direct or indirect cause of all diseases is due to lack of fiber in our regular diet.

Under this situation, we have no other alternative than to introduce the crude medicines Bio-Herbs for treatment of all chronic diseases. In fact treatment of all complicated diseases like cancer, HIV, arthritis, diabetes, cardiovascular disease, etc. remains "incomplete" without extensive application of crude medicines. It has been acknowledged by scientists all over the world that the so-called "refined medicines" have certain limitation to achieve smooth cure. They are now recommending daily intake of 20-35 grams of dietary fiber, whereas we are far behind the requirement.

New path of treatment:

Not depending on patients' likings, satisfaction or taste we therefore, recommend Bio-Herb Nos. 1 & 2 for universal application irrespective of disease. These herbal medicines will provide you abundant dietary fiber to counterbalance environmental pollution from water, air, microwaves and above all food pollutions (adulterated and junk-foods) which you cannot avoid in modern civilization. Medicines will also provide you plenty of natural vitamins, minerals and Biochemic ingredients.

Conclusion:

We should not blame blindly the system which is responsible for evil effect of pollution (i.e. modern civilization), but our ignorance to fight against pollution should be first criticized. Considering pollution is inevitable in modern civilization, we should have awareness to fight the same by medicine. Fiber-enriched Bio-Herbs are the special instrument to fight against the pollution by direct means. Additionally, we have Bio-Tone Plus and Booster medicine to increase the efficiency of internal glands and organs to support the detoxification schema.

DIETARY FIBER WILL KEEP YOU HEALTHY AND PRACTICALLY DISEASE-FREE. IF TAKEN REGULARLY, IT WILL DEFINITELY INCREASE YOUR LONGEVITY BY AT LEAST 5 YEARS!

---

*   *   *

CHLOROPHYLL AND COLOURED PIGMENTS THE LIFE FORCE OF HEALTH

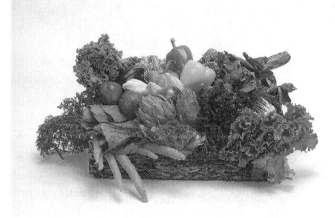

The greatest curse of our modern civilization is the rapid increase of complicated diseases like cardiovascular disease, diabetes, neurological disease, cancer and AIDS. Instead of going deep into genetic factors, we will concentrate our attention on the basic reason or the underlying cause of the disease. Advancement of civilization has lead to destruction of forests i.e. plants, herbs, trees and flowers. Rapid industrialization in 20th century has practically disturbed ecological balance with profound change in lifestyle and food habit. Environmental pollution due to industrialization and modernization of agriculture with extensive use of chemical fertilizer, harmful pesticide and genetically modified food are the matter of concern for major health hazards and spread of serious diseases, especially in urban areas.

Hence it is evident that the more we are going away from Nature, the more increase of diseases are observed. We are 100% dependent on Nature to utilize the "useful solar energy" to convert the same into chemical energy, heat energy and mechanical energy to maintain our body function. The reason is, unlike plant we do not have Chlorophyll in our body and therefore, we have to depend on conventional foods for nutrition. It is the only plants which convert "useful solar energy" into "chemical energy" in the form of carbohydrates, proteins and fats. In fact all animals, including carnivorous animals depend on plants (chlorophyll) directly or indirectly.

Chlorophyll and coloured pigments form the building-block of life. Green plants are rich in chlorophyll whereas coloured fruits, vegetables and flowers are the main source of 'natural coloured pigments'. Go to any forest and look at the Nature—you will discover the vibrant of colours in Nature. Green leaves and multicoloured fruits, vegetables and flowers form the beauty of Nature. Plants and trees in the forest never fall sick—thrive hundreds or few thousand years combating with scorching sunshine, thunders, storms and other natural calamities. Lesson is if you want to remain healthy, beautiful and disease-free, you must be aware of the amazing power of chlorophyll and coloured pigments. Though not recorded in textbooks, some of its magnificent benefits on health are indicated below:

1) Normal activity can be maintained with very low calorie (about 500 Kcal per day), if sufficient amount of green chlorophyll is taken from fresh leaves, vegetables and fruits. This means transfer of pure solar energy stored in chlorophyll is so efficient that we can easily forget our textbooks where requirement is stated as 2000 to 2500 Kcal per day.

2) Role of coloured pigments available in Nature (termed as Bioflavonoid, Beta carotene, etc.) is simply beyond our imagination. In presence of chlorophyll, bioflavonoid helps to develop immune system of the body, enhances activity and functioning of Immunoglobulin, corrects metabolic disorder, eradicates formidable diseases like heart disease, diabetes, asthma, obesity, neurological disorder, cancer and even some of the genetic diseases.

We especially highlight these wonderful aspects of green chlorophyll and coloured pigments for maintenance of health. In fact you need not take any medicine if you are habituated in taking natural chlorophyll and bioflavonoid. Teach your children the importance and function of these two pigments so that they can give-away taking medicine in their life.

Unfortunately, property and structure of chlorophyll and bioflavonoid are greatly lost due to the process of cooking. In fact these should be taken in purest form i.e. in un-cooked condition in the form of juice, salad, etc. For treatment of serious diseases like cancer, we recommend intake of plenty of chlorophyll and coloured pigments available from coriander leaves, *tulsi*, *neem*, carrot, black grapes, apple, orange, watermelon, pineapple, coloured non-toxic flowers such as *jaba*, rose, etc. through juice or salads, over and above intake of medicines.

Life-force or Bio-force thus greatly depends on the green and coloured natural pigments. Though we are proud of advancement of science, "Life Force" still remains mysterious, but time will come when it will be regarded as "Fundamental Force" in Nature and will be recognized by the scientists all over the world.

TAKE PLENTY OF CHLOROPHYLL AND COLOURED PIGMENTS IN ALL COMPLEX DISEASES TO ACHIEVE FASTEST CURE IN SHORTEST TIME.

KEEP AWAY DISEASE BY USING THESE "NATURAL MEDICINES"

---

*   *   *

MEDICINE, DIET AND EXERCISE

SOME SPECIAL FEATURES

Our system of treatment (Biopathy) calls for special attention on Medicine, Diet and Exercise. Based on these three main pillars of treatment, most of the chronic and complicated cases which are difficult to cure by conventional system can be cured in the easiest way.

MEDICINE

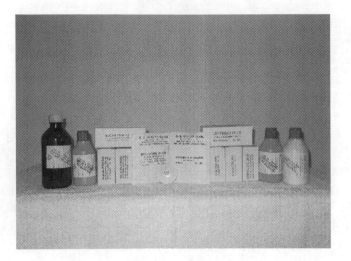

We have limited number of medicines for treatment of chronic diseases. Medicines are absolutely free from any side-effect whatsoever. These are applicable to child as well as old, medicines have "multipurpose" and "multifarious" functions—activates internal organs and system e.g. liver, lung, heart, kidney, stomach, pancreas, uterus, nervous system, blood and circulatory system, excretory system, reproduction system, etc. Most important feature of our medicine is that it detoxifies the whole body by removing accumulated toxins of the body, caused by environmental pollution and incorrect food habit. Besides, the medicine caters for maintenance of health of Eye—the most important organ responsible for mental peace and stability.

Salient features of application of medicines:

Medicines are extremely useful to correct "metabolic disorder" irrespective of disease. In fact most of the chronic disease is the outcome of "metabolic disorder" of the whole body i.e. disharmony of nervous system, lymphatic system and circulatory system—it may be cold and cough, tonsillitis, arthritis, high or low pressure, high cholesterol, skin disease, hypothyroidism, hyperthyroidism, fatty liver disease, etc. In fact we need not break our head to find out medicine for individual disease—simply by improving of "metabolic function" the patient can get relief in shortest way.

Remedies to correct Metabolic Disorder:

i) For glands and internal organs: Bio-Tone Plus and Booster ii) For Liver function: Sugar-Tablet or Liv-Treat and Shakti-Raj iii) For Detoxification: Bio-Herb Nos. 1 & 2 iv) For protection of saliva, gum and supplementing magnesium. Danta-Raj herbal toothpowder v) For Bio-Energy required for mitochondria: Green Chlorophyll and Coloured Pigments (bioflavonoid) from Nature and lastly vi) For maintenance of Skin and Eye: Multi-Care or Aqua-Fresh and Herbal Eye-Drop respectively. All these medicines will complete the process of cure.

If medicines are continued for lifelong patients will get rid of complicated disease and avoid surgery in life. Remember, toxins are accumulated everyday in the body and we need to expel the same on regular basis.

It has become easy to treat little babies and children because medicines are non-toxic in all respect and we need not think too much for selecting the remedy—in fact there is no question of overdosing. Repeat the medicine as per intensity of the disease.

DIET

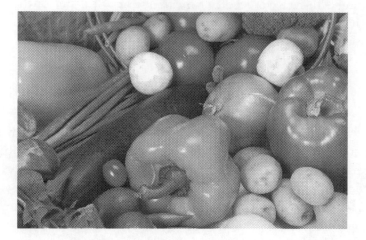

Depending on the intensity and complication of the disease, take Green Chlorophyll and Coloured Pigments (bioflavonoid) daily from green and coloured leaves, vegetables, fruits and non-toxic coloured flowers. Needless to say, these pigments are destroyed during cooking or by exposure to excessive heat or cold. In fact useful Solar Energy or Bio-Energy is stored in green and coloured pigments, which directly influence Chromosome or Gene and vitalizes mitochondria of the living cell. This useful solar energy (Bio-Energy) is the internal energy of every living object of our Planet and this energy can be termed as "Life Force".

Under green pigment coriander leaf, cucumber, guava, green peas etc. are very useful. Patients suffering from diabetes, heart disease and cancer must take plenty of green leaves in un-cooked condition. Under coloured pigment vegetables, carrot, tomato, orange, apple, black grape, watermelon, pineapple, etc. are easily available. These green and coloured pigments are essentially required for the patients of arthritis, skin disease, heart disease, diabetes and specially cancer—in fact they cannot be cured without these pigments.

Avoid animal protein as far as practicable, especially from the age of thirty. One must be aware of the fact that excessive animal protein in our daily diet is one of the leading causes of incurable diseases like cardiovascular disease, arthritis, diabetes, cancer and even AIDS. In fact human anatomy and genetics are not very suitable for intake of animal-protein enriched diet. Therefore restriction of animal protein in our daily diet must be considered to be of *high importance* for maintenance of health as well as treatment of diseases. Take more vegetable-protein by reducing animal-protein from your diet.

Those who desire to heal their troublesome disease within a short time; they should stop taking conventional diet (rice or wheat) for one or two weeks or reduce to minimum. They need to take diet of green and coloured vegetables such as carrot, apple, banana, black grapes, watermelon, etc. all in un-cooked condition and mix with some cooked vegetables or milk for taste.

Alternatively, patients must take sufficient amount of Bio-Herbs (Bio-Herb No. 1 & 2) to expel accumulated toxins from the body. Take plenty of these herbs before going to bed or in the morning. Take sufficient water in the morning in empty stomach. The accumulated toxins will come out of body through soft or semi-liquid stool. The process of expelling toxins from body is called detoxification.

Patients suffering from chronic disease should take more alkaline food to balance acid-alkali pH. In fact we are diseased because we consume more acidic food than alkaline food. It is interesting to know that intake of raw-garlic and 10-15 pieces of green *neem* leaves daily in empty stomach in the morning and with plenty of water can keep away many diseases in life. Therefore we should make habit of taking raw-garlic and green *neem* leaves daily for maintenance of health on long term basis.

EXERCISE

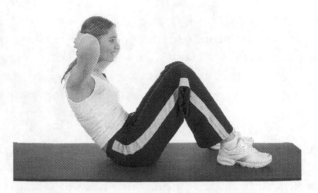

Light or moderate exercise of any type is very much useful for maintenance of health. Walking for about half an hour daily in the morning should be practiced. Heavy or vigorous type exercise is not considered to be beneficial in the long run. We recommend exercise for those people who are able to do so. Breathing exercise ('Deep Breathing' and 'Fast Breathing') is effective in most of the diseases, especially in asthma or sinus. For diabetic patients fast-walking, jogging or running proves to be very effective.

However, people of heart disease should consult doctor before doing vigorous exercise. Patients of arthritis may need special exercise—Physiotherapy or Electrotherapy.

Meditation is also considered to be a form of exercise. It reduces irregular pulses generated in our brain due to mental stress of our busy and modern lifestyle. Meditation can restore normal activity of brain and helps to reduce all types of psychosomatic diseases. Practicing meditation is especially recommended to prevent diseases like attention disorder, Alzheimer's disease and many other neurological diseases.

> ## KEYWORD OF BIOPATHY SYSTEM OF TREATMENT IS "MEDICINE, DIET AND EXERCISE"

*   *   *

CHAPTER-2: MEDICINE

BIO-TONE PLUS (TRIPLE STRENGTH)

MEDICINE FOR ALL DISEASES

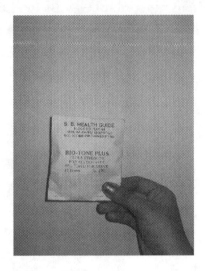

It is a wonderful multifarious type of medicine for application in all diseases and has highest curative action. Bio-Tone Plus and Booster medicines are mainly of Ayurvedic with Biochemic preparation, and complementary to each other. In most of the disease, these two medicines are generally used in 2:1 ratio, which means Bio-Tone Plus is normally used twice the quantity of Booster medicine. However, in nerve-related disease, Bio-Tone Plus and Booster should be taken in 3:1 ratio to exhibit the best effect.

Bio-Tone Plus has profound capability of influencing nervous system, lymphatic system and blood or circulating system, thereby brings balance or harmony between the three. Disease is caused due to imbalance of above systems; hence application of Bio-Tone Plus (in combination with Booster) is compulsory for all types of acute and chronic disease. General and special application of Bio-Tone Plus are as follows:

Nerve-related disease:

Neurological diseases such as acute and chronic vertigo, Parkinson's disease, migraine, epilepsy, headache, eye and optic-nerve related diseases, flashing sensation of nerves, pain due to sciatica and arthritis, erratic type pains, severe or shooting pain anywhere in the body, weakness of memory especially at old age, attention disorder, schizophrenia, insomnia, Alzheimer's disease, psychiatry disorder, general debility of Nerves and so on.

Lymph-related disease:

Diseases due to deficiency of immunity system of the body such as viral fever, influenza, tendency to get cold, tonsillitis, pharyngitis, bronchitis, pneumonia, bacterial and fungal infection, endocrine diseases like diabetes, hypothyroidism and hyperthyroidism, fatty liver disease, gastritis, chronic constipation, weakness of digestion, swelling of lymph glands and even malignant diseases like cancer and tumour.

Blood-related disease:

High cholesterol, high or low blood pressure, heart diseases like angina pectoris, food allergy, dust allergy, bleeding piles, fistula, eczema, psoriasis, boils and abscess, eosinophilia, liver disorder, toxin-related diseases like environmental pollution, fever due to attack of virus, bacteria, parasites, etc.

Bio-Tone Plus (Double Strength):

Triple strength of Bio-Tone Plus is having highest range of curative action especially on neurological problems (e.g. migraine, Parkinson's disease, sciatica, vertigo, etc.), lymph-related diseases or immunity disorder (e.g. swelling of glands, tonsillitis, bronchitis, fatty liver disease, diabetes, cancer, etc.) and should be universally applied from practical point of view.

Bio-Tone Plus of "Double Strength" is having comparatively low curative value. Therefore, "Triple Strength" must be applied in all complicated diseases to achieve best result.

Always remember Bio-Tone Plus (Triple Strength) for any type of acute and chronic disease related to "head", "nervous system" and "glands". Blindly apply "Triple Strength" of Bio-Tone Plus alternated with Booster in all diseases—majority of diseases will be cured within shortest period of time.

*   *   *

BOOSTER

MEDICINE FOR ALL DISEASES

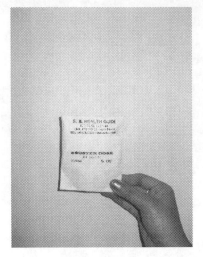

It is a complementary medicine of Bio-Tone Plus. The medicine is also of multifarious type in its action and has profound curative power. Medicine should be applied to all diseases in combination with Bio-Tone Plus. Booster is also a powerful medicine to bring harmony between nervous system, lymphatic system and circulating system, similar to Bio-Tone Plus mentioned above.

APPLICATION OF BIO-TONE PLUS AND BOOSTER FOR TREATMENT OF ALL CHRONIC AND COMPLICATED DISEASES

Bio-Tone Plus and Booster medicines are considered to be the most effective for treatment of all complicated diseases. Medicines contain little amount of ayurvedic *swarna* and *roupya bhasma*—thereby eradicating "*tridosha*". Though costly compared to other medicines, their range of action is simply outstanding. These medicines are having wide range of action, act on nerves, muscle, bone, blood and all internal organs such as liver, heart, kidney, eye and so on. Few examples of special application of these two medicines in chronic as well as acute diseases are separately mentioned below.

DISEASES WHERE BIO-TONE PLUS (TRIPLE STRENGTH) AND BOOSTER TO BE APPLIED

A)	**NERVE-RELATED AND IMMUNITY DEFICIENCY DISEASES** **Preferred Ratio of Bio-Tone Plus and Booster: 3:1**
•	Neurological and Head-related Disease (Central and Peripheral Nervous System): Acute Vertigo, Severe Migraine, Parkinson's Disease, Writer's Cramp, Sciatica, Erratic Pain of Nerves, Flashing Sensation, Shooting or Pulsating Pain anywhere in the body, Headache, Brain Tumour, Weakness of Optic Nerves of Eyes.
•	Nerve-related Heart Disease: Sick Sinus Syndrome, Irregular Pulse, Sinus Bradycardia, Tachycardia, Sino-arterial Block.
•	General Psychiatry Problems (applicable for non-violent and co-operative type patients): All types of Psychiatry disorders e.g. Depression, Dementia, Fear, Weakness of Memory, Schizophrenia, Alzheimer's Disease.
•	Allergy and Immunity Deficiency: Dust Allergy, Food Allergy, Recurring Cold and Cough.
•	Disease of Respiratory System: Severe Bronchitis with High Fever, Pneumonia, Cold and Cough, Chronic Asthma.
•	Geriatric or Old Age Disease: General Health Problem in Old Age, Weakness of Nerves, Shortfall of Memory, Chronic Bronchial Problems, Weakness of Digestion.

•	**Tonic for Maintenance of Health:** General Health Tonic for all, Health Tonic for Children and Pregnant Mother, Avoidance of Surgery in Life, Leading Disease-free Life, Increase of Longevity.
•	**SUGGESTED DOSE:** 1) Starting dose: Say 2 doses Bio-Tone Plus and 1-2 doses Booster daily for 2-3 months. 2) Maintenance dose: Say 1-2 doses Bio-Tone Plus daily for 20 days and 1 dose Booster daily for 10 days in a month. It is better to continue the medicine lifelong.
B)	**LYMPH-BLOOD RELATED DISEASES** **Preferred Ratio of Bio-Tone Plus and Booster: 2:1 or 1:1**
•	Disease of Digestive System—Acidity, Piles, Fistula: Chronic Acidity, Gas, Weak Digestion, Weak Liver, Chronic Dysentery, Constipation, Bleeding Piles, Fistula.
•	Liver-related Heart Disease: High or Low Blood Pressure, High Cholesterol, High LDL, Coronary Artery Disease (CAD), High-grade Tonic for Heart.
•	Arthritis and Bone-related Disease: Chronic Arthritis, Joint Pain, High Uric Acid, Gout, Osteoporosis, Fluoride Poisoning.
•	Disease of Lymph and Endocrine Glands: Swelling and tenderness of Glands, Hypothyroidism, Hyperthyroidism, Fatty Liver Disease, Jaundice, Enlargement of Liver, Obesity.
•	Skin Disease: Itching, Eczema, Urticaria, Psoriasis, Recurring Boils & Pimples, Arsenic Poisoning.

•	<u>Female Disease:</u> Menstrual Pain, Leucorrhoea, Excessive Bleeding, Menopause problem, Uterine and Breast Tumour.
•	<u>High Fever, Severe Cold and Cough:</u> Severe Tonsillitis, Pharyngitis, Flue, Running Nose, Viral Fever, Unknown type of Fever, Throat Irritation, Cold and Cough.
•	<u>SUGGESTED DOSE:</u> 1) Starting dose: Say 1-2 doses Bio-Tone Plus and 1-2 doses Booster daily for 2 3 months. 2) Maintenance dose: Say 1-2 doses Bio-Tone Plus daily for 20 days and 1 dose Booster daily for 10 days in a month. It is better to continue the medicine lifelong. 3) For high-fever & severe throat infection start high doses of medicine as per "Special Points" below.
C)	**NERVE-LYMPH-BLOOD RELATED DISEASES** **Preferred Ratio of Bio-Tone Plus and Booster: 2:1 or 1:1**
•	<u>Destructive type Disease:</u> Cancer—Treatment as well as Preventive measure. Diabetes (Type-2) or Blood Sugar, Diabetic Neuropathy.
•	Start high doses of medicine as per "Special Points" referred below. Requirement of medicine is several times more than normal patients.

SPECIAL POINTS ON APPLICATION OF BIO-TONE PLUS AND BOOSTER:

Infants and babies	=	Lactating mother should take Bio-Tone Plus and Booster themselves. Infants will be medicated through mother's milk. Alternatively, give "Fever-Cold" and "Stomach-Stool" which are equally effective for babies.

Severe or acute condition	=	In case of high fever, tonsillitis, severe throat infection, bronchitis, severe cold and cough, shooting or pulsating pain anywhere in the body, take repeated or multiple doses of Bio-Tone Plus and Booster on the very first day (say 4-5 doses medicine of each type). Thereafter take maintenance dose.
Cancer and Diabetic patients	=	Disease being of destructive type, requirement of Bio-Tone Plus and Booster is several times more (say 3-4 doses Bio-Tone Plus and 2-3 doses Booster daily) than the normal patients. Thus the cost of treatment in Cancer or Diabetes is much higher than normal disease. Fix-up the dose depending on the severity of disease.
Alternate the medicine daily?	=	You need not alternate the medicine frequently. Initially take both the medicines daily for a month or so. Thereafter, take the medicines in your own style. Consume certain amount of medicine on monthly basis. Note that even if you take medicine in most irregular way it will work!
What is the "Minimum Dose" of medicine?	=	Dose referred in the book corresponds to higher-grade of problems, because all patients do not have same intensity of problem—some may have lower grade and some higher grade. It may be noted that sometimes only few doses are sufficient to get rid of the ailment, if medicines are taken immediately at beginning of the problem. Therefore, it is important to apply the medicine at the time of onset of the problem.
When and how long to continue medicine?	=	Take medicine anytime i.e. in full-stomach or empty-stomach or half stomach. Medicines are deep acting—it will act on all conditions. It is better to continue the maintenance dose of medicine for lifelong. Best medicine for maintenance of health of aged people.

BIO-TONE PLUS + BOOSTER	=	• HEAD AND NERVE RELATED DISEASE • GLAND AND LIVER RELATED DISEASE • LUNG RELATED DISEASE • HEART AND BLOOD RELATED DISEASE	• AVOID OLD AGE DISEASE • AVOID SURGERY IN LIFE • BE DISEASE-FREE • INCREASE LONGEVITY • TAKE MAINTENANCE DOSE, SAY 1-2 PACKETS BIO-TONE PLUS AND 1 PACKET BOOSTER IN A MONTH

GENERAL RULE FOR DOSES OF BIO-TONE PLUS AND BOOSTER	=	DOSE SHOULD BE SUCH THAT MEDICINAL FORCE BECOMES EQUAL TO THE DISEASE FORCE. THUS, STARTING DOSE MAY BE SEVERAL TIMES HIGHER THAN NORMAL MAINTENANCE DOSE. NOTE THAT THERE IS NO QUESTION OF OVERDOSING BECAUSE THERE IS NO SIDE EFFECT EVEN IF YOU TAKE LARGE AMOUNT OF MEDICINE.

IN CASE OF ACUTE PROBLEM, APPLY REPEATED DOSES OF BIO-TONE PLUS (Triple) AND BOOSTER AT 15-30 MINUTES INTERVAL, TILL THE CRISIS PERIOD IS OVER. IF THE CASE IS NOT SURGICAL, YOU WILL GET IMMEDIATE RESPONSE.

APPLY BIO-TONE PLUS AND BOOSTER IN ALL COMPLEX DISEASES—IT WILL COVER ABOUT 60% OF TOTAL MEDICATION VALUE. FOR DETAIL REFER TABLE-I

APPLY BIO-TONE PLUS AND BOOSTER TO YOUR CHILD CONTINUOUSLY FOR 2-3 YEARS. THEY WILL BE PRACTICALLY FREE FROM 80% OF DISEASE.

*　*　*

"SHAKTI-RAJ" HEALTH TONIC

FOR CHILDREN, ADULT AND OLD

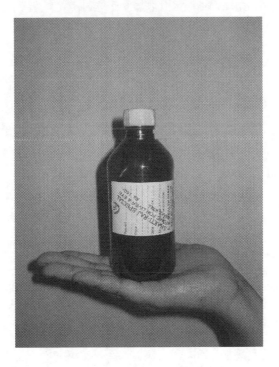

An important tonic used in almost all ailments of liver, digestive system and eye. It is prepared especially in combination with pure and natural honey, which also provides vital nutrients to the people of all ages—children, adults and old. Following are the main application of Shakti-Raj:

General Application:

Used in chronic acidity and indigestion, heartburn, rumbling feeling and heaviness of stomach, tenderness in the region of liver. Effective in cleaning of blood, reduces uric acid, cholesterol, pain on joints and muscles, gout, osteoarthritis, bleeding piles and fistula. Improves blood-circulation and prevents formation of clots in the blood. Remedy is indicated in all types of skin disease, formation of recurrent boils and carbuncles, cardiovascular diseases, varicose vein, weakness of liver and heart, eye diseases. If taken regularly, it can reduce risk of malaria and mosquito-borne diseases. It helps to prevent even cancer and tumour, if taken regularly for the whole life. Special application of the medicine is given below:

Tonic for growing children:

Medicine contains high grade Calcium, Magnesium, Phosphorous, Zinc and Vitamin B-complex and therefore, considered essential for growth and development of intelligence of especially school-going children.

Tonic for old people:

Old people generally suffer from sluggishness of digestive system and nerves (geriatric problems). For them Shakti-Raj along with Bio-Tone Plus, Booster and Sugar-Tablet or Liv-Treat is ideal.

Tonic for eye, especially glaucoma:

Function of optic nerve improves, if taken regularly. Shakti-Raj is a compulsory medicine for glaucoma for lowering the eye-pressure.

Tonic for arthritis, CVD and diabetes:

It is a high grade tonic for arthritis, especially for the patients suffering from high uric acid. An invaluable tonic for weakness of heart, reduces bad cholesterol (LDL) and triglyceride. Because of its honey or fructose content, it marginally lowers the blood sugar level (around 5%) for the patients of diabetes.

Tonic for Fatty Liver Disease:

It is a compulsory medicine for treatment of fatty liver disease. The fructose content in the medicine is invaluable to improve the function of liver.

Tonic for Summer:

It cools down the body in summer or hot-weather and brings comfort. Take 3-4 caps medicine regularly in summer to reduce the possibility of heat-stroke.

Direction of use:

Take 1-2 caps Shakti-Raj (honey mixed) and 5-6 Sugar-Tablet or Liv-Treat tablets immediately after food, once or twice daily (at breakfast, lunch or dinner). These two medicines are complimentary to each other, improve digestive power and help assimilation of nutrients from food.

For any type of chronic and complicated disease, add Bio-Tone Plus, Booster and Bio-Herb in your list of medicine.

Shakti-Raj may be taken directly or mixed with little water to reduce the feeling of sour taste which may not be liked by all persons.

It is better to continue the medicine for the whole life.

**AN EXCELLENT TONIC FOR GROWING CHILDREN.
PROTECTS BODY FROM SUMMER AND HOT WEATHER.
ENSURES IMPROVEMENT OF LIVER FUNCTION.
A COMPULSORY MEDICINE FOR TREATMENT OF
GLAUCOMA AND EYE DISEASE.**

---

*   *   *

"SUGAR-TABLET" AND "LIV-TREAT"

HERBAL TABLET WITH BIOCHEMIC MEDICINE FOR DIGESTIVE SYSTEM

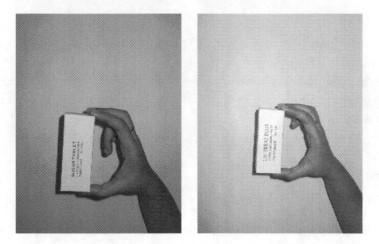

Herbal tablet blended with essential Biochemic medicines, for treatment of all diseases related to liver, digestive system, blood and skin. Following are the main application of Sugar-Tablet or Liv-Treat:

Main Application:

It is indicated in all types of stomach problems such as chronic acidity, indigestion and gas for many years. Medicines are especially effective in chronic and acute dysentery, amebiasis, bleeding piles and all types of skin disease such as eczema, itching of skin, recurring boils and carbuncles, etc. Purifies blood, reduces LDL cholesterol and triglyceride of the blood.

If taken with Shakti-Raj, it reduces uric acid and chronic arthritic pain. It is especially indicated in all types of Jaundice. It is a high grade tonic to improve the function of liver.

Direction of Use and Remark:

Take 5-6 tablets along with 1-2 caps Shakti-Raj immediately after food, once or twice daily (at breakfast, lunch or dinner). For children, dose may be 1-2 tablets. Taste of the tablet is bitter—swallow it with water.

Sugar-Tablet or Liv-Treat will help to neutralize acidic taint of the food taken by increasing pH value and converts the food to relatively alkaline (pH > 7 is alkaline, pH < 7 is acidic) in nature (note that alkaline food is ideal for the body). Sakti-Raj on the other hand, helps assimilation of nutrients from the digested food. Sugar-Tablet or Liv-Treat and Shakti-Raj are thus complimentary to each other—these medicines are the supporting pillar to correct the "metabolic disorder". Continue these two medicines for whole life.

Note that though action of both medicines is almost same, Sugar-Tablet is more powerful than Liv-Treat. Sugar-Tablet is equally effective for both diabetic and non-diabetic patients. For diabetic patients it moderately reduces blood-sugar level.

> **BOTH SUGAR-TABLET AND LIV-TREAT ARE EXCELLENT MEDICINES FOR LIVER. MEDICINES PURIFY BLOOD AND KEEP RESULTANT FOOD RELATIVELY ALKALINE.**

> **SUGAR-TABLET IS ESSENTIAL FOR BOTH DIABETIC AND NON-DIABETIC PATIENTS. IT REDUCES RISK OF BEING DIABETIC. ALSO REDUCES TENDENCY OF CHRONIC DYSENTERY WHICH IS A COMMON PROBLEM OF PEOPLE LIVING IN TROPICAL CLIMATE.**

*   *   *

"BIO-HERB" MEDICINES

BIOCHEMIC-MIXED HERBS FOR DETOXIFICATION

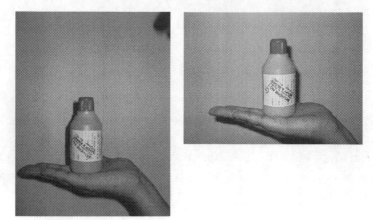

These are important herbal medicines for treatment of all types of chronic diseases and for better functioning of internal organs of the body. Two types of Bio-Herbs are available—BIO-HERB No. 1 and BIO-HERB No. 2, for general and multipurpose use. Both types of Bio-Herbs are blended with Biochemic medicines and are the richest sources of "natural vitamins" and "dietary fibers".

Bio-Herb No. 1 works better for "Heart and Blood". It improves function of heart, purifies blood, and reduces LDL Cholesterol and Triglyceride from the blood. Bio-Herb No. 2 works better for "Liver and Kidney". These two medicines are essential for treatment of all diseases such as constipation, chronic cold and cough, acidity and gas, arthritis, uric-acid, fatty-liver disease, thyroid, obesity, cardiovascular disease, diabetes, skin disease and so on.

Thus combination of Bio-Herb Nos. 1 & 2 protects the vital organs and the whole body. Continuous use of these medicines will ensure protection from all types of complex disease, especially cardiovascular diseases. "Bio-Herbs" are the wonderful medicines to correct

"Metabolic Disorder" and are the best answer for prevention of dreadful diseases like Cancer and AIDS.

These medicines not only provide "natural vitamins" but also supplement basic nutrition of the body. It protects the body from toxins and environmental pollutions, helps to maintain good health. These medicines must be used in all diseases to speed-up the process of cure.

Bio-Herbs should be taken regularly by sick as well as healthy people of all ages irrespective of disease. These medicines have plenty of "dietary fiber" and hence, excellent for "Detoxification of the Body". For treatment of any complex and multiple diseases, take plenty of Bio-Herb 1 or 2 at bedtime and drink sufficient water in empty stomach in the morning—toxins like arsenic, fluoride, pesticide, etc. will come out of your body through soft or liquid stool. Regular intake of Bio-Herb medicines will surely increase longevity of people by at least five years.

CURE IS NOT EXPECTED IN COMPLEX DISEASES WITHOUT INTAKE OF SUFFICIENT DIETARY FIBER ON REGULAR BASIS. APPLY BIO-HERBS IN ALL COMPLEX DISEASES TO ACHIEVE WONDERFUL RESULT.

BIO-HERBS ARE THE ONLY MEDICINES FOR RAPID DETOXIFICATION AND EXPEL TOXINS ACCUMULATED IN YOUR BODY FROM ENVIRONMENTAL POLLUTION (ARSENIC, FLUORIDE, PESTICIDE AND CHEMICAL POLLUTIONS).

BIO-HERBS ARE THE EXCELLENT MEDICINES FOR PURIFICATION OF BLOOD. MEDICINES WILL PROTECT YOU FROM DREADFUL DISEASES.

---

*   *   *

"DANTA-RAJ" HERBAL TOOTHPOWDER

MEDICINE FOR MULTIPURPOSE ACTION AND ORAL HYGIENE

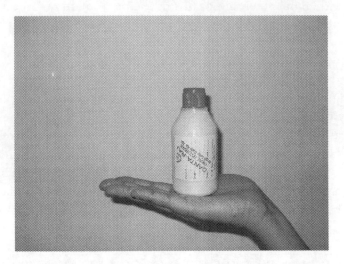

Danta-Raj, a marvelous bacteria-destructive herbal toothpowder, is used in various problems like pyorrhea, offensive odour in mouth, swelling of gum, toothache, oozing of blood from gum, sore in mouth and tongue, spongy gum, etc. If tooth becomes loose in childhood due to some reason, use it—tooth will be stronger. It is incomparable in keeping mouth clean and fresh. If care is taken harmful bacteria cannot take entry into stomach—as a result disease can be prevented, especially stomach trouble. It prevents mouth cancer—as no chemical mixed with it, gum become strong and root of tooth remains strong.

Remember, it is desirable to keep tooth intact at the age of even 70-75 years—thus the body can be protected from complex diseases. It is compulsory for the patients of diabetes, high-pressure and arthritis to use fluoride-free Danta-Raj herbal toothpowder. This toothpowder is also economic in all respect. It is better to brush teeth twice daily (morning and night). In case of high blood-sugar or formation of cavity on teeth, treatment of diabetes or dental surgery is needed.

<u>Tonic for nerves and digestive system:</u>

Danta-Raj is magnesium-based herbal toothpowder—it is a high-grade medicine for general maintenance of health. It supplements magnesium in the body, the deficiency of which causes many diseases, especially debility of nerves.

It is a wonderful tonic to keep the optic nerves lively, eyesight better— it prevents all types of eye diseases, if regularly used from childhood.

It has got beneficial action on digestive system. During treatment of all chronic or complex diseases, it is mandatory to use Danta-Raj to improve the efficiency of the digestive system. Brush teeth using Danta-Raj toothpowder and apply Multi-Care lotion on your gum and swallow the medicine—you will be surprised to note that one-third of your stomach problem has been diminished.

Always use hard quality brush to clean your teeth by Danta-Raj. Store the medicine in cool place—do not expose to heat or sun for long time.

EASIEST WAY TO PREVENT ALL DENTAL PROBLEMS IS TO KEEP YOUR MOUTH AND GUM HEALTHY.

AVOID FLUORIDE POISONING

Use DANTA-RAJ Herbal Toothpowder twice daily at Morning and Night. **Brush application.**	**Apply few drops MULTI-CARE Lotion on your Gum and massage for few minutes and then swallow the medicine (lotion is also helpful to reduce your stomach problem). Apply at least twice or thrice in a week.**

> **STRONG TEETH AND HEALTHY MOUTH INDICATE STRENGTH OR POWER OF YOUR BODY. TIGERS AND LIONS ARE CONSIDERED INVALID ONCE THEIR TOOTH STARTS LOOSENING!**

> **DANTA-RAJ IS A HIGH-GRADE MULTIPURPOSE MEDICINE. REGULAR USE OF THIS IS THE BEST WAY TO PREVENT ORAL-CANCER.**

*   *   *

"MULTI-CARE" POWERFUL ANTISEPTIC AND PAIN-RELIEVING HERBAL LOTION

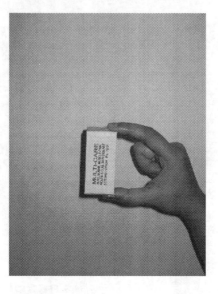

Multi-Care is a wonderful multifarious herbal lotion having profound antiseptic, antibacterial, antifungal and anti-inflammatory action. Medicine acts on multiple areas—it is used for internal as well as external application. It is for multipurpose use, hence an essential item for all family.

Antiseptic action:

It is a powerful antiseptic lotion for application in all types of cuts and wounds. Medicine will stop bleeding and prevent formation of pus. It is a high-grade antiseptic lotion for healing of the wounds. In case of excessive bleeding, apply cotton soaked with medicine and then bandage the area.

Relieves severe muscle pain:

Medicine works wonderfully to relieve all types of pain due to injury of the muscle. It quickly subsides inflammation and swelling (except pain due to fracture of bone). Just apply few drops of medicine on the painful area and rub gently with your finger. In case of excessive pain, apply several times.

Skin-care lotion:

It is extremely useful in all types of ulcer, severe itching on folds of skin, eczema, abscess, boils, carbuncles, bleeding and wounds, painful tumour on skin, itching and swelling of piles with feeling of rawness. The lotion is ideal for application on the tender skin of infants and babies.

Dental and mouth care:

The lotion works marvelously in all types of dental problems such as severe toothache, swelling, bleeding and softening of gum, pyorrhea, loosening of teeth due to injury, ulcer on gum, mouth and tongue. Used for protection of gum and saliva. For strengthening or hardening of gum, apply few drops on gum and gently rub by finger.

Diarrhea, vomiting and dysentery:

In case of severe diarrhea, vomiting or abdominal pain due to bacillary dysentery or cholera, mix 5-6 full droppers of above medicine with 8-10 caps of Shakti-Raj in a glass of water and drink slowly—finish the mixture within half an hour or so. You will be surprised to get relief of above problems within a short time.

Miscellaneous:

The medicine also works well in all types of digestive problems e.g. acidity, gas, stomach-ulcer, etc.—therefore when you apply it for strengthening of gum, swallow the medicine. Partial benefit is found in tingling cough, tonsillitis, throat pain and sciatica.

Multi-Care is a concentrated variety of antiseptic herbal lotion, whereas "Aqua-Fresh" is diluted variety of the same medicine. Where quick result is to be obtained within a short time, apply 'Multi-Care' lotion.

MULTI-CARE IS A HIGH GRADE MEDICINE FOR WIDE RANGE OF APPLICATION—CUTS, BURNS, MUSCLE PAIN, ULCER & ITCHING ON SKIN, SWELLING OF GUM, ETC.

BRUSH YOUR MOUTH TWICE DAILY BY DANTA-RAJ TOOTHPOWDER. APPLY FEW DROPS MULTI-CARE LOTION ON YOUR GUM—RUB AND THEN SWALLOW THE MEDICINE. MOUTH WILL BE BACTERIA-FREE AND YOU WILL GET RID OF ONE-THIRD OF YOUR STOMACH PROBLEMS.

---

*   *   *

NON-IRRITANT TYPE HERBAL "EYE-DROP"

FOR ALL EYE DISEASE & PROTECTION FROM ENVIRONMENTAL POLLUTION

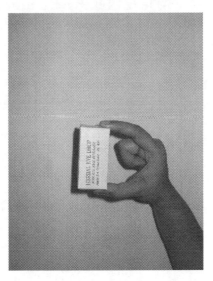

The herbal Eye-Drop is completely non-irritating and useful in all types of eye disease like conjunctivitis, eye sore, stye, myopia, optic atrophy, night blindness, glaucoma, Eale's disease, corneal disease, vitreous opacity and so on. It is useful to everybody—elderly or children.

It prevents all types of complications like eyes of computer worker, excessive watching of T.V., air pollution, microwave and electromagnetic pollution, even increasing of eye power and progress of cataract.

Eye Care with General Maintenance of Health:

Eye-Drop is to be used in all cases of eye disease especially school and college students regularly. For chronic eye disease treatment with internal medicine as well as external medicine (eye-drop) is essential and proves to be most effective. Thus, along with it use magnesium based Danta-Raj herbal toothpowder for keeping optic nerves lively. Besides, take Bio-Tone Plus, Booster, Shakti-Raj and Sugar-Tablet or Liv-Treat on regular basis. For constipation and to expel toxins from body, take plenty of Bio-Herbs. Take herbal bath of Aqua-Fresh for benefit of the eye. All these medicines will work internally not only on eyes, but also on other diseases like gastritis, weakness of liver and digestion, constipation, piles, skin disease, asthma, diabetes, high pressure, high cholesterol, arthritis, allergy, cold and cough, throat pain and tonsil, thyroid, tumour, and female diseases.

Importance must be given on Eye Care for flourishing memory and intelligence of children. Do not store the eye-drop for long period—use fresh bottle.

However the same result is obtained by mixing 10-15 drops Multi-Care lotion or 3-4 droppers Aqua-Fresh in a glass or cup of water and then washing eyes with the mixture. It is interesting to note that some people find this method of application more convenient than the standard eye-drop. Direct application of 1 or 2 drops Multi-Care or Aqua-Fresh on eyes is also recommended as an alternative to eye-drop. Thus you can totally eliminate Home-stock medicine of herbal eye-drop (also refer Table-X).

AN IDEAL HERBAL "EYE-DROP" FOR LIFELONG USE. PROTECTS EYE FROM ENVIRONMENTAL POLLUTION. TAKE BIO-TONE PLUS, BOOSTER AND SHAKTI-RAJ AS INTERNAL MEDICINE FOR TREATMENT OF ALL EYE DISEASES.

---

*　　*　　*

"AQUA-FRESH" HERBAL BATH ANTISEPTIC AND ANTIFUNGAL LOTION-CUM-COSMETIC

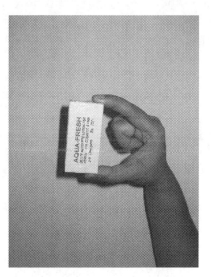

Usefulness of Aqua-Fresh herbal bath is of three fold. Firstly, in skin care or cosmetic use it is unrivaled. Secondly, it gives benefit if applied in any skin disease, itching on folds of skin, etc. Thirdly, we get some comfort if applied on the painful area of the muscle. It works like Multi-Care, but being a diluted variety, its curative power is comparatively less.

It is effective after-bath herbal lotion for skin. Removes micro-particles of soap used during bath and the skin becomes smooth. Keeps skin healthy and retards aging effect or wrinkling of the skin. It has excellent antiseptic, antibacterial and antifungal action on skin. Removes tiredness and brings freshness and comfort after bath. It is an ideal lotion for herbal bath of small babies. It is also an excellent and ideal cosmetic for ladies. It is an excellent antiseptic after-shaving lotion.

Remember, for maintenance of children's health, Bio-Tone Plus, Booster and Aqua-Fresh herbal bath are essential.

High-grade Cosmetic:

For skin care or for cosmetic application, those who spend plenty of money in cosmetics, they can spend minimum using Aqua-Fresh, which is of high standard. Everybody knows that by application of conventional beauty creams, the pores or sweat-glands of the skin get blocked by sticking small particles of dust from air. On the other hand skin can easily soak Aqua-Fresh medicine—as a result for its influence, bad odour of body goes away, skin becomes soft and cool—even skin disease cures.

Aqua-Fresh is also an excellent remedy for prevention of hair-fall caused due to dandruff.

High-grade Skin-care for infants:

For infants and small babies, mix few droppers Aqua-Fresh (or few drops Multi-Care) in Olive Oil and massage the whole body. The herbal antiseptic medicine will work wonderfully on the tender skin of babies.

Direction of use:

After bath pour 3-4 full droppers of medicine in small quantity of water and mix properly—then pour it on all parts of the body. Removes micro particles of soap from body—moreover it will make skin soft and lively. During the herbal bath, small particles of medicine will touch all parts of the body, covered or uncovered. As spray painting is better than brush painting, likewise herbal bath is better than all other systems of skin care. Thus body is benefited—especially it is better, ideal and scientific for protection of skin of the small children by Aqua-Fresh from dust and bacteria.

Important Note:

Aqua-Fresh is only a dilute variety of Multi-Care lotion. It can be substituted by Multi-Care for all practical purpose. By keeping Multi-Care under Home-stock medicine, one can totally eliminate requirement of Aqua-Fresh.

PROTECT YOUR BABIES FROM ANY TYPE OF SKIN INFECTION BY USING AQUA-FRESH HERBAL LOTION. HIGH GRADE COSMETIC FOR SKIN AND HAIR-CARE.

---

*   *   *

"SONALI" POWERFUL ANTISEPTIC HERBAL CREAM

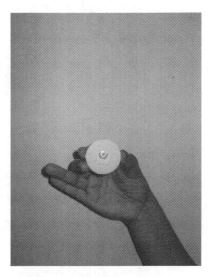

Sonali works wonderfully in any type of bleeding from cuts and wounds, burns, bites of poisonous insects such as bees, wasps, etc.

Antiseptic cream:

It is a powerful antiseptic for any type of cut form sharp instrument, as well as after-shaving application. Apply the cream—bleeding will be stopped immediately. In case of deep cuts with excessive bleeding, apply the medicine with cotton and bandage the area. To eradicate all possibilities of "tetanus" take 3-4 droppers 'Fever-Cold' liquid medicine 2-3 times daily for a week.

It is an essential item for children who are often affected by cuts.

Bites of poisonous insects:

It relieves pain and burning sensation from bites of poisonous insects such as bees, wasps, etc. Apply on the painful area—you will get immediate relief.

Burns from spillage of hot oil, etc.:

Apply immediately on the affected area of the skin—no blister will come out. It is an essential item for housewives who are often affected by burns during cooking. Always keep the medicine in your kitchen.

Skin-care cream:

It is an ideal and high-grade cosmetic for cracks on feet or skin. Wash your feet at night and apply the cream—you will get wonderful result. It moderately works in boils, carbuncles, dry eczema and skin disease, barber's itch, etc.

Sonali is an ideal cream for First-aid management. This medicine is used for external application only and should not be applied on eyes or tongue.

> ### MULTI-CARE IS ALSO A "POWERFUL ANTISEPTIC LOTION" FOR ALL TYPES OF CUTS AND BURNS. APPLY WHICHEVER IS AVAILABLE IN YOUR HAND.

* * *

STANDARD LIQUID MEDICINES FOR COMMON USE—SPECIAL APPLICATION FOR CHILDREN FEVER-COLD MEDICINE

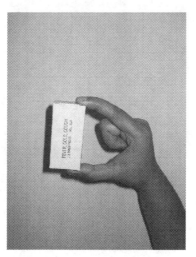

It takes care all types of fever and especially useful for the children. During onset of fever, flue or running nose, take medicine repeatedly at 10-15 minutes interval till fever subsides. In case of fever with stomach problem, alternate this medicine with 'Stomach-Stool'. This medicine is having excellent anti-tetanus and anti-allergic property. It cools down the excitement of nerves.

It must be however, noted that the medicine works well in simple type of fever, cold and cough. But in case of complicated cases like swelling of tonsils, bronchitis or fever of unknown type with severity, always apply repeated doses of 'Bio-Tone Plus' and 'Booster' in combination (generally in 2:1 or 1:1 ratio). Thus you can practically eliminate Fever-Cold medicine from Home-stock (also refer Table-X).

STOMACH-STOOL MEDICINE

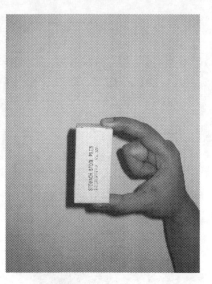

Medicine takes care of all types of stomach problems such as indigestion, rumbling of stomach, diarrhea of many types, vomiting, bleeding of piles, etc. In case of feeling of uneasiness in stomach, take this medicine repeatedly at 15-20 minutes interval. It is an essential remedy, especially for children.

However, in case of severe diarrhea with vomiting like cholera, it is better to take a mixture of 'Multi-Care' and 'Shakti-Raj'. Read "Crisis Management" mentioned in this book. For chronic acidity and gas, generally Sugar-Tablet proves to be more effective than Stomach-Stool.

> **BOTH MEDICINES ARE COMPLEMENTARY TO EACH OTHER. ONE MEDICINE PARTLY COVERS AREA OF THE OTHER. APPLY WHICHEVER IS AVAILABLE WITH YOU.**

> FEVER-COLD AND STOMACH-STOOL CAN COVER ALMOST ALL DISEASES OF INFANTS AND CHILDREN. HOWEVER, TO INCREASE IMMUNITY POWER OF YOUR CHILDREN, APPLY BIO-TONE PLUS AND BOOSTER ON REGULAR BASIS.

*   *   *

KEEP READY STOCK OF MEDICINES WITH YOU FOR FAMILY TREATMENT

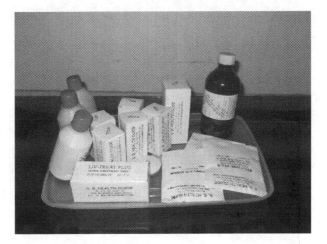

We do not treat patients with large number of medicines. All medicines are having multifarious actions. Most of the diseases, except surgical cases and high-grade genetic disorders, can be cured with these limited numbers of medicines by blind application of the same. Use of only few medicines eliminates confusion of the treatment. The medicines are thus called user-friendly and family-medicine.

On the topmost position we have Bio-Tone Plus (Triple Strength) followed by Booster medicine. These two medicines have profound capability to protect all internal organs, glands and nerves and have potentiality to correct high-grade metabolic disorder. Irrespective of disease, these two medicines can be safely applied to small children, adults and very old persons.

Next we have "General medicines" i.e. Sugar-Tablet or Liv-Treat, Shakti-Raj, Bio-Herb (Nos. 1 & 2), Danta-Raj herbal toothpowder and non-irritating herbal Eye-Drop to correct the metabolic disorder. We have high-grade antibacterial, antifungal and pain-relieving herbal lotion Multi-Care and antiseptic herbal cream Sonali. Lastly we have Aqua-Fresh, a high-grade antibacterial and antifungal herbal cosmetic for maintenance of skin, especially for infants, children and ladies.

Medicines are aimed for not only to cure diseases, but also to maintain overall health of your family members. Use daily these medicines as health tonic and replace the deficient stock periodically. Another point is that medicines do not expire even though you keep the same for few years (except for Eye-Drop). For a medium-size family following medicines are normally suggested for ready home-stock:

Essential Medicines Suggested for Family-stock:

1)	Bio-Tone Plus 'Triple Strength' (for all diseases)	:	6-8 Packets
2)	Booster (for all diseases)	:	4 Packets
3)	Sugar-Tablet or Liv-Treat (tablets of bitter taste)	:	1 Phial each
4)	Shakti-Raj (health tonic for all ages)	:	1 Bottle
5)	Bio-Herb No. 1 (herbs and biochemic)	:	2-3 Bottles
6)	Bio-Herb No. 2 (herbs and biochemic)	:	2-3 Bottles
7)	Danta-Raj (herbal toothpowder)	:	2-3 Bottles
8)	Multi-Care (antiseptic and pain-relieving herbal lotion)	:	1 Phial
9)	Sonali (herbal antiseptic cream)	:	2-3 Pieces

Remember:

Aqua-Fresh and Herbal Eye-Drop can be totally replaced by a single medicine Multi-Care. Use 1-2 droppers Multi-Care during herbal bath or for cosmetic purpose. Apply 1-2 drops Multi-Care directly on eyes during eye-disease (like conjunctivitis) or wash eyes by diluting the medicine in water. Therefore Aqua-Fresh and Eye-Drop are not included under list of essential medicines for Home-stock.

Optional Medicines Suggested for Family-stock:

1)	Stomach-Stool (liquid medicine)	:	1 Phial
2)	Fever-Cold (liquid medicine)	:	1 Phial
3)	Aqua-Fresh (herbal bath and cosmetic)	:	1 Phial
4)	Herbal Eye-Drop (or replace by Multi-Care or Aqua-Fresh)	:	1 Phial

For maintenance of health, 1 packet each Bio-Tone Plus and Booster may be consumed in a month by each of your family members. These medicines are of high-grade tonic for health. Let the medicines be consumed by your school-going children as well as very old members of your family. Consumption of medicines for diseased persons or patients is however, more than above requirement. Bio-Tone Plus and Booster will cover up the major area of problems. However, other "General medicines" as listed above should also be utilized by your family members, because the medicines have got special role of action. Therefore, all medicines are equally important for overall maintenance of health.

Take special care of your children so that they do not become victim of complicated disease when they become adult or old. By this way you can reduce total expenditure on treatment by not having complicated disease and also by avoiding surgery and hospitalization, for which you may have to spend bulk amount of money. Always it is better to start your home-treatment at "Zero" hour without wasting time for searching medicine or visit us (doctor) for advice. Take care of your health by supplementing advanced type of health-tonic-cum-medicine. Remember the old proverb: "Prevention is better than cure". Hence, a little awareness on health will definitely save your money as well as time.

IMPORTANT NOTE:

Variety of Home-stock medicines can be further reduced by knowing the difference between "Basic or Primary medicines" and "Derivatives or Secondary medicines". Refer "Table-X" and note that the number of medicines under Home-stock can be practically reduced to only 7 or 8 instead of 13 medicines listed above. It is up to you to use reduced variety of Home-stock medicines.

> **FAMILY-STOCK WILL PREVENT YOU FROM ALMOST ALL DISEASES INCLUDING HOSPITALIZATION.**

* * *

ALWAYS CARRY ESSENTIAL MEDICINES IN TRAVELER'S KIT DURING YOUR FAMILY-TOUR

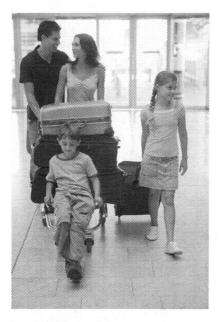

When you travel with your family, it is of utmost importance to keep yourself and your family members free from health-hazard. Due to change in weather, your child may suffer from viral fever, tonsillitis, cold and cough, throat pain, etc. It is not guaranteed that you will take bacteria-free water and food all the time. Especially people of plain dry land are not accustomed with the drinking water of the tropical coastal region and therefore, there is risk of stomach problem like amebiasis, dysentery and indigestion.

Whatever may be situation, a simple way of prevention of disease will make your tour happy and peaceful. Just before one or two days of your journey, start taking 1 dose each Bio-Tone Plus and Booster daily till you complete your tour. These two medicines will definitely elevate your immunity level to a great extent and you will be practically free from unwanted problems due to change of weather. Always carry few packets of Bio-Tone Plus and Booster with you.

Take 5-6 Sugar-Tablet or Liv-Treat tablets and 1-2 caps Shakti-Raj daily during meals to keep your stomach trouble-free. These medicines will also relieve threat from mosquito-borne disease, if taken continuously from one month before your tour. Take plenty of Bio-Herb to eradicate constipation due to change of food-habit during your tour.

Apply Multi-Care (alternatively Aqua-Fresh) antiseptic-cum-antibacterial lotion or Sonali antiseptic cream immediately on any type of cuts and wounds or muscle pain due to injury. In case of severe diarrhea (watery stool) with or without vomiting, mix 5-6 full droppers of Multi-Care medicine with 8-10 caps Shakti-Raj in a glass of water. Consume the mixture within a short time. Repeat this process once or twice as applicable. You will be surprised to realize that searching for doctor is not necessary. Alternatively, take repeated dose of Stomach-Stool till the stomach trouble becomes normal.

Thus by using multifarious type of medicines, you will be absolutely free from tension during your whole tour. Keep all the useful medicines in your briefcase to encounter the unwanted problems which may arise during your tour.

Emergency management:

It must be remembered that Bio-Tone Plus has profound capability to control certain emergency situations like severe vertigo, unbearable pain of nerves anywhere in the body, pain due to rheumatoid arthritis, severe headache and migraine, severe throat infection or bronchitis or tonsillitis with high-fever and so on. Under these situations apply Bio-Tone Plus repeatedly; say at 15-30 minutes interval, with few doses of Booster medicine. In most of the cases, you will find that your crisis period gets over within few hours.

Suggested Medicines for Traveler's Kit during long tour:

1) Bio-Tone Plus (Triple Strength) and Booster   : 6-8 Packets each

2) Sugar-Tablet or Liv-Treat and Shakti-Raj   : 1 Phial each

3) Bio-Herb Nos. 1 & 2 (herbs and biochemic)   : 1 Bottle each

4) Stomach-Stool (liquid medicine)   : 4 Phials

5) Danta-Raj (herbal toothpowder)   : 1 Bottle

6) Multi-Care (antiseptic and anti-inflammatory : 1 Phial
   herbal lotion)

7) Sonali (antiseptic cream)   : 1 Piece

BUSY PROFESSIONALS OR LADIES SHOULD ALWAYS CARRY 1 PACKET EACH BIO-TONE PLUS AND BOOSTER (WEIGHING ONLY FEW MILLIGRAMS) IN THEIR BRIEFCASE OR VANITY BAG.

---

*   *   *

CHAPTER-3: TREATMENT OF DISEASES

TREATMENT OF NEUROLOGICAL DISEASES

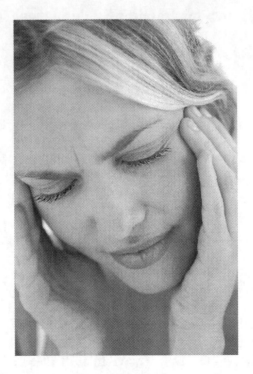

Bio-Tone Plus and Booster are the wonderful medicines for all types of neurological diseases. The action of these medicines is to supply nutrition to the nerves. Thus treatment of neurological disease is very much simplified—one need not scratch his head to find out the reasons or underlying causes of neurological disorders. Simply apply the medicines to get the desired result. Medicines work smoothly on nervous system, lymphatic system and circulatory system to restore their normal functions. Note the simplified treatment of few complicated neurological disorders:

VERTIGO: SEVERE AND CHRONIC TYPE

Brilliant cure is achieved for any type of positional vertigo—mild or severe. Depending on the severity, take 1-2 doses Bio-Tone Plus and 1 dose Booster daily for 3-4 months. However, the starting dose may be increased depending on the severity. It is better to continue the medicine for a year.

Additionally take General medicines (Sugar-Tablet or Liv-Treat, Shakti-Raj, Bio-Herb and Danta-Raj) for overall improvement of your system.

MIGRAINE, ERRATIC NEUROLOGICAL PAIN, SEVERE HEADACHE

Do you believe that chronic Migraine of many years can be cured easily within a few months? Erratic neurological pain or problems such as sensation of sudden pain at different organs or parts of the body can be cured smoothly? Headache form unknown reason (not related with eye or spectacle problem) can be relieved by simple treatment? Initially take 1-2 doses Bio-Tone Plus and 1 dose Booster daily, for 3-4 months—thereafter continue the maintenance dose. You will be relieved from the unwanted or peculiar problems within a year or so.

Use General medicines (Sugar-Tablet or Liv-Treat, Shakti-Raj, Bio-Herb and Danta-Raj) to accelerate the process of cure.

Always remember "Bio-Tone Plus" for any type of "Nerve-related Pain"—it may be severe headache, arthritic pain, injury of muscle and so on. Apply the medicine repeatedly in shooting or pulsating pain occurring anywhere in the body.

PARKINSON'S DISEASE, WRITER'S CRAMP

Miraculous cure is observed by taking Bio-Tone Plus and Booster continuously for about a year. Initially take 2-3 doses Bio-Tone Plus and 1 dose Booster on regular basis for 2-3 months. Thereafter, dose may be reduced to 1-2 doses Bio-Tone Plus and 1 dose Booster daily.

Take supportive medicines (Sugar-Tablet or Liv-Treat, Shakti-Raj, Bio-Herb and Danta-Raj) to correct metabolic disorder. Intake of green chlorophyll and coloured pigments (bioflavonoid) of nature in the form of leaves, vegetables, fruits and non-toxic coloured flowers proves to be very useful.

It is better to continue all medicines for whole life for keeping you fit, since Parkinson's disease or writer's cramp is generally found in people of old age.

Exercise and physiotherapy in combination with internal medicines is more helpful for treatment of Parkinson's disease.

FLASHING SENSATION OF NERVES, SEVERE AND SHOOTING PAIN OF NERVES, SCIATICA

Instead of scratching your head to find out the cause of flashing sensation of your nerves, or searching for suitable remedy for sciatica, just take Bio-Tone Plus and Booster. Take 1-2 doses Bio-Tone Plus and 1 dose Booster daily and continue the medicines for 2-3 months. In case of specific neurological pain (say flashing pain on gum), additionally apply 'Multi-Care' concentrated herbal lotion or 'Aqua-Fresh' dilute lotion on the affected area.

Take General medicines (Sugar-Tablet or Liv-Treat, Shakti-Raj, Bio-Herb and Danta-Raj) for overall maintenance of health.

EPILEPSY, BRAIN-FAG, BRAIN TUMOUR, AFFECTION OF BRAIN, BED WETTING OF CHILDREN

All these diseases are due to weakness or over-excitement of nerves. Bio-Tone Plus and Booster are the leading remedies for all types of problems related to brain or nervous system. Initially start with 2-3 doses Bio-Tone Plus and 1 dose Booster daily for 3-4 months. Thereafter, the dose may be reduced to 1-2 doses Bio-Tone Plus and 1 dose Booster daily, depending on the situation. In case of sudden problem, repeated dose of 'Fever-Cold' or 'Stomach-Stool' liquid medicines may prove to be effective.

It is essential to take General medicines (Sugar-Tablet or Liv-Treat, Shakti-Raj, Bio-Herb and Danta-Raj) for improvement of metabolic activity.

OLD AGE PROBLEMS: PREVENT MEMORY LOSS, ALZHEIMER'S DISEASE, WEAKNESS OF NERVES

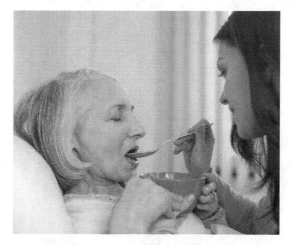

Majority of old people suffer from bronchial problems, cardiovascular disorders, stomach problem, arthritis and weakness of nerves resulting in shortfall or even loss of memory. Moreover, people at old age slowly become resistant to the common drugs—as a result it becomes extremely difficult to cure respiratory problems such as chronic cold and cough, bronchitis, pneumonia etc. Take 1-2 doses Bio-Tone Plus daily with one-third quantity Booster medicine on regular basis throughout the year. By this way your immunity will not only increase but also weakness of nerves, shortfall of memory, neurological problems like Alzheimer's disease, Parkinson's disease, etc. will be within your control. It is better to continue the medicines for rest of your life.

Additionally, take General medicines (Sugar-Tablet or Liv-Treat, Shakti-Raj, Bio-Herb and Danta-Raj) for maintenance of health. These medicines will also definitely reduce all types of old age problems (geriatric diseases).

VISION AND OPTIC NERVES: EASY METHOD FOR GIVING UP SPECTACLES

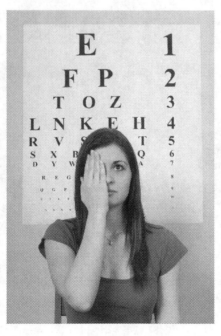

Bio-Tone Plus, Booster and Shakti-Raj are high-grade tonic for optic nerves. Besides, magnesium-based herbal toothpowder Danta-Raj is extremely useful for optic nerves. Vision of eye, especially for children and teenagers greatly improves with better functioning of optic nerves.

It is interesting to know that majority of children and youngsters having moderate range of power can easily give up spectacles by improving the efficiency of optic nerves. Take 1-2 doses Bio-Tone Plus daily and half the quantity Booster for 1-2 years. Additionally take Shakti-Raj and Sugar-Tablet or Liv-Treat daily with food, brush your teeth with Danta-Raj toothpowder and apply Herbal Eye-Drop on your eyes on regular basis. Check your vision every 6 months interval—you will be sure to get improvement of your eyesight. Replace your existing spectacle immediately after improvement and get accustomed with the reduced power.

Above simplified process of giving up the spectacles is successful in most of the cases for children and youngsters.

80% CHILDREN AND YOUNGSTERS CAN GIVE UP WEARING SPECTACLES! JUST TRY AND GET WONDERFUL RESULT.	=	TAKE 1-2 DOSES BIO-TONE PLUS AND 1 DOSE BOOSTER DAILY FOR 1-2 YEARS. TAKE SHAKTI-RAJ AND SUGAR-TABLET OR LIV-TREAT AND USE DANTA-RAJ. APPLY HERBAL EYE-DROP REGULARLY.
WEAR GLASSES OF SLIGHTLY LOW POWER THAN ACTUALLY RECOMMENDED. CHECK EYESIGHT ON EVERY 6 MONTHS. DEPENDING ON THE PROGRESS, STOP WEARING SPECTACLES WHEN YOUR EYE-POWER COMES DOWN TO ± 1.0 OR LESS		

PSYCHIATRIC DISORDERS, PSYCHOSOMATIC DISEASES

Underlying causes of psychiatry diseases are self and environmental disorder triggered by socio-economic structure of the modern age. In other words constitutional factor (genetic taint) and social factors like unit-family structure, excessive psychological stress on students as well as professionals, problem of loneliness especially in old age, etc., are the root cause of mental imbalance or psychiatry disorders. Bad effects of mind are transmitted to the body—as a result list of psychosomatic diseases are increasing day by day. Presently many of the diseases like peptic ulcer, ulcerative colitis, anorexia, hypertension, bronchial asthma, impotence, frigidity, menstrual disorders such as amenorrhea, dysmenorrhea, menorrhagia and diseases like urticaria, psoriasis, eczema, diabetes, rheumatoid arthritis, migraine, etc., are known to of psychosomatic in origin.

It may be noted that majority of the patients do not show any violence; hence do not require sedative drug. If the patient is non-violent and shows co-operation by taking our medicines sincerely, one can expect steady improvement or control of the disease. Take 1-2 doses Bio-Tone Plus daily and one-third the quantity Booster on regular basis to achieve the best result. The medicine may be continued throughout the life in 3:1 or 2:1 ratio (Bio-Tone Plus vs. Booster).

It is important that General medicines (Sugar-Tablet or Liv-Treat, Shakti-Raj, Bio-Herb and Danta-Raj) be taken for overall improvement. In addition to above, counseling by Psychologists may be helpful for critical and complicated cases.

Treatment of violent and non-supportive type patients is not under the scope of our treatment.

*   *   *

TREATMENT OF DISEASES FOR LYMPH AND ENDOCRINE GLANDS

Lymph glands and lymph nodes play the most significant role in defensive mechanism or immunity system of the body. There are 500-600 lymph glands distributed throughout the body—it is the function of these glands by which the immune cells (lymphocytes) develop. These glands are the primary sites of defensive barrier to spread of illness such as infectious diseases, cancer, etc. Enlargement or malfunction of glands signifies illness of the body. Swelling of tonsils, pharyngitis, hypo or hyper thyroidism, spread of cancer—all have relevance to the functional deficiency of lymph glands.

Endocrine glands such as pineal gland, pituitary gland, thyroid gland, adrenal gland, liver and pancreas, kidney, ovary and testis, are closely related with lymph glands. These glands secret hormones or associated with information signal network like hormones. We observe hormonal imbalance of body, when secretion from endocrine glands is in excess (hyper) or less (hypo). Often we find tumours growth (benign or malignant) of these glands.

Function of lymph glands and endocrine glands are complementary to each other—in fact function of one is dependent on the function of the other. In true sense all diseases ranging from simple fever or flue to serious and destructive diseases like Diabetes, Cancer, Tumour and AIDS—all are the outcome of functional disturbance of lymph and endocrine glands which is broadly termed as "immunity disorder" or "metabolic disorder". In fact all serious and complicated diseases are due to metabolic disorder—therefore, it is better to correct the "metabolic disorder" to achieve fruitful result.

Suggested method of treatment for diseases related to disorder of lymph nodes and endocrine glands are discussed below.

TREATMENT OF CANCER, BREAST AND UTERINE TUMOUR, ETC.

Cancer is categorized as destructive disease (like diabetes)—toxins spread gradually from the place of origin to the other parts of the body through the lymph nodes, which is the producer of immunity or lymphatic cells as well as carrier of waste or toxin. While treatment of cancer by genetic manipulation is of remote possibility, our treatment is based on conservative method only, by correcting the immune system of the body or metabolic disorder.

Bio-Tone Plus and Booster are effective remedy to take care of metabolic disorder. The requirement of dose depends on the severity of disease and varies from person to person—one may initially need large doses like 2-3 doses Bio-Tone Plus and 1-2 doses Booster 2-3 times in a day (i.e. total 10-12 doses) to counterbalance the disease force. Dose may be reduced after 2-3 months, depending on the improvement.

Supportive medicines for cancer must be taken regularly to correct the "metabolic disorder":

- Shakti-Raj and Sugar-Tablet or Liv-Treat, to be taken twice daily with food and continue for whole life. These two medicines will reduce the cancerous tendency of the patient.
- Bio-Herb No. 1 or 2, to be taken plenty for direct detoxification of toxins as well as supplementing "natural vitamins" and "dietary fiber".
- Danta-Raj fluoride-free herbal toothpowder twice daily (brush application) for supplementing magnesium in the body.
- Diet of plenty of green chlorophyll and coloured pigments (bioflavonoid) available from green leaves, coloured vegetables, fruits and non-toxic coloured flowers, to be taken daily in empty stomach. For detail refer "Recommended Diet for Cancer Patients".

- Take less or minimum protein (especially animal protein) and plenty of vegetables to make your resultant diet less acidic in nature.

By meticulously following above treatment, one can resist spread of cancer through lymph glands which is considered as the most important aspect of the treatment.

* * *

TYPICAL CHART OF MEDICINE AND DIET FOR CANCER PATIENTS

HOMEOPATHY MEDICINES:

Arsenicum alb. 30—When pain is indicated. Take on SOS basis.

Carcinocin in milicimal step-up potency—Subsides pain and stops progress of cancer.

Coffea 30—When sleep is impaired.

Lacasis 30—When problems are mainly indicated in the morning after getting up from sleep.

Sulpher 30—Problems aggravate at midnight, patient likes sweet foods.

Calcaria carb 30—Mainly for women patients of flabby constitution.

Other medicines like Phosphorus 30, Thuja oc. 30, Asteries rubens 30, Symphytum 30, Psorinum 200, etc. may be taken symptomatically.

Medicines will work only if totality of symptoms of the patient tallies with particular medicine.

Alternatively:

Take standard medicines "Fever-Cold" or "Stomach-Stool" liquid, instead of searching for matching homeopathic medicine.

AYURVEDIC MEDICINES:

Bio-Tone Plus (Triple Strength) and Booster—These are the most important medicines covering nervous system, lymphatic system and circulatory system. Dose of the medicine is to be decided as per virulence of the disease, some patients may need large doses of medicine, say 2-3 doses Bio-Tone Plus and 1-2 doses Booster 2-3 times in a day (total 10-12 doses). Initially large doses of medicines prove to be very much effective—after 2-3 months, dose may be reduced depending on the improvement. Maintenance dose of medicines should be continued for whole life.

Shakti-Raj and Sugar-Tablet or Liv-Treat—Medicines function especially on liver and regulate bile for digestive system. Take 2-3 caps Shakti-Raj and 6-8 Sugar-Tablet or Liv-Treat tablets daily after food (breakfast, lunch or dinner). Shakti-Raj is an anti-cancerous remedy. Both medicines have good effect on liver.

Bio-Herb Nos. 1 & 2—These medicines will remove constipation, help direct detoxification and keep the body-function all right. Take plenty—as much as you can, say 4-5 spoons daily. It can be taken at bedtime and also in the morning with sufficient water to expel toxins from the body. Additionally take 3-4 glasses of juice of green chlorophyll and coloured pigments in empty stomach.

Danta-Raj and Herbal Eye-Drop—It is compulsory to brush with Danta-Raj herbal toothpowder for keeping mouth bacteria-free and supplementing magnesium in body. Apply herbal eye-drop twice daily for protection of eyes from air pollution, microwave radiation, etc.

Aqua-Fresh Herbal Bath—It is always better to take herbal bath by using Aqua-Fresh—the medicine will prevent infection of skin due to bacteria or fungus.

Multi-Care herbal antiseptic lotion—Toxins of Cancer spread through lymph nodes distributed all over the body. Thus, cancer patients in general, face problem of swelling of glands in any part of the body. During swelling, the patients feel pain on the region—apply above medicine on the painful area to subside the pain. In case of non-availability of this medicine—apply Aqua-Fresh, which will also help to subside the pain, however to a lesser extent.

RECOMMENDED DIET FOR CANCER PATIENTS:

Foods of low nitrogen-content will be best suited. Low nitrogenous foods are carbohydrates. Avoid protein especially animal protein as far as practicable. Take plenty of vegetables. Take 2 chapattis each at breakfast, lunch and dinner—with sufficient vegetables and *Dal*. Note that light food like *Khoi* in Bengali is preferred instead of chapatti at the time of dinner.

Never eat full-stomach meal or dinner. Keep half or one-third of your stomach empty. Instead of taking more food, take more fruits and vegetables.

Green Chlorophyll and Coloured Pigments:

Take plenty of juice of fresh coriander, *pudina* or similar type of leaves of green plants, leaves of wheat, lettuce, pumpkin, etc.; 1-2 full glass of juice daily, at morning in empty stomach. Sometimes juice of *Gulancha* proves to be helpful. Take some amount of carrot, *dalim*, black grapes, watermelon, apple, tomato, pineapple or similar type of coloured fruits or vegetables, daily either in the form of salad or in the form of juice made in juice-making machine. Take 2-3 full glasses of the juice of coloured fruits in the morning in empty stomach, at least 1 hour before taking food. Slowly add some *Tulsi*-leaves or *Jaba*-flower or rose-flower in the above juice to enhance the quality of juice.

For cancer patients it is of high importance to take above mentioned juice from fresh green leaves, vegetables, coloured fruits and non-toxic coloured flowers to supplement Bio-energy (Bioflavonoid) to the mitochondria of cells.

It is better to give-up conventional breakfast in the morning by taking 3-4 full glasses of mixed juice of green and coloured pigments, all in empty stomach. Note that one should avoid taking fruits or juice just after meals. Patients should also take at least 15-20 pieces of fresh green *neem* leaves, few non-toxic coloured flowers and raw-garlic for whole life.

This type of treatment also proves to be extremely helpful for the patients of Diabetes, because both of the diseases are of destructive type, which need large amount of chlorophyll and bioflavonoid for better functioning of the lymph glands.

TREATMENT OF CANCER	=	START HIGH DOSES OF BIO-TONE PLUS AND BOOSTER DAILY.	+	ADDITIONALLY TAKE GENERAL MEDICINES (SUGAR-TABLET OR LIV-TREAT, SHAKTI-RAJ, BIO-HERB & DANTA-RAJ)	+	IT IS COMPULSORY TO TAKE 1-2 GLASSES OF JUICE OF GREEN LEAVES + 2-3 GLASSES OF JUICE OF COLOURED FRUITS IN EMPTY STOMACH IN THE MORNING

REFER TABLE-I FOR COMPARATIVE EFFECT OF VARIOUS MEDICINES FOR TREATMENT OF CANCER.

*   *   *

TREATMENT OF FOOD ALLERGY AND DUST ALLERGY

Allergy is primarily a disorder of immune system of the body. Immunoglobulin is produced by lymphatic network of the body and duly activated and controlled by the nerve-signaling system of the brain. Persons who are allergic to various foods or dust show hypersensitivity disorder through antigen-antibody reaction from dust or specific food items like prawn, brinjal, ladies-finger, milk, etc. In case of food allergy, rash-type swell and round come out of skin and virulent type itching sensation is experienced in the affected area. In case of dust allergy, patients suffer from sneezing, watery discharge from nose and feeling of rawness inside the nostril.

Take 1-3 doses of Bio-Tone Plus daily and half quantity Booster on long term basis to build up specific immunity against the antigen. However in case of sudden and violent attack of the problem such as rash on skin or repeated sneezing, take Bio-Tone Plus and Booster frequently, say 3-4 doses of each type daily. Very often during attack, repeated doses of 'Fever-Cold' also subsides the problem of itching and feeling of rawness of the nose.

Initially allergic people should avoid the allergens or the items from which they are affected. After treatment for 3-4 months, they should make habit of consuming small quantity of the prohibited foods periodically.

By this process one can slowly become immune to food or dust allergy. Remember, allergy is a metabolic disorder of high-grade and needs to be treated for few years to achieve complete cure.

*   *   *

TREATMENT OF HYPOTHYROIDISM AND HYPERTHYROIDISM

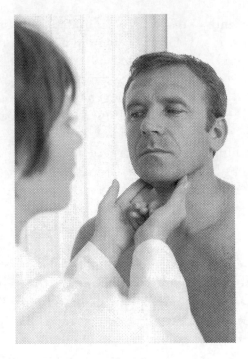

The thyroid gland produces T3 and T4 hormones which are important in regulating general metabolism. These hormones are important to increase oxygen consumption and modulate the development process. Insufficient amount of free thyroid hormones result in the condition known as hypothyroidism and characterized by slow heart rate, diastolic hypertension, sleepiness, constipation, sluggish behavior, sensitivity to cold, dry skin and hair, and a sallow complexion. In hyperthyroidism excess hormones are produced by the thyroid glands resulting rapid heart rate, inability to sleep, nervousness, excessive sweating, weakness, and moist skin.

Take 1-2 doses Bio-Tone Plus and 1 dose Booster daily for at least six months or a year. Additionally take Sugar-Tablet or Liv-Treat, Shakti-Raj and plenty of Bio-Herbs (No. 1 & 2) for 'natural vitamins' and 'dietary fiber'. Take sufficient green chlorophyll and coloured pigments (bioflavonoid) available in nature from fresh green leaves, coloured vegetables, fruits and non-toxic coloured flowers.

Test for T3, T4 and TSH after 4-6 months and check the status of improvement.

*   *   *

TREATMENT OF OBESITY OR WEIGHT GAIN

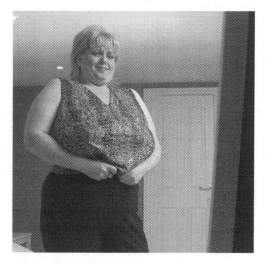

Obesity is considered to be foundation of many diseases like arthritis, high cholesterol, high pressure, diabetes, fatty liver disease, thyroid, infertility and so on—one may suffer from one or many diseases above mentioned. Generally habit of overeating, taking junk and un-hygienic food, lack of 'natural vitamins' and 'dietary fibers' and leading sedentary life are the main cause of obesity and gaining of weight—however in some cases genetic taint predominates.

Treatment of reduction of fat:

Though in true sense obesity depends on fat cell count of the body, the tendency to grow obese can be minimized by correcting the food habit along with intake of medicines for 'metabolic disorder'. Bio-Tone Plus and Booster are the important remedies for correction of lymphatic system, especially the lymph nodes. Take 1-2 doses Bio-Tone Plus and 1 dose Booster daily at least for one or two years. Medicines may however be continued for whole life, if desired.

Additionally take plenty of Bio-Herbs (4-5 spoons daily) to detoxify your system. This will also provide you 'natural vitamins' and 'dietary fibers', which are essential to retard the process of accumulation of fat. Besides, to correct the liver-function, take regularly Sugar-Tablet or Liv-Treat and Shakti-Raj along with the food once or twice daily. Brush with Danta-Raj herbal toothpowder to supplement magnesium in your body.

For obese people, it is essential to take low calorie but energetic diet. Take plenty of green chlorophyll and coloured pigments (bioflavonoid) such as raw juice of coriander leaves, green leaves of wheat, lettuce leaves, carrots, pineapple, watermelon and different types of fruits and non-toxic coloured flowers. Juice of pumpkin (*Lau* in Bengali or *Lauki* in Hindi or *Dudhi* in Marathi) prevents accumulation of fat to a great extent. It is better to give up conventional breakfast by taking few glasses of above juice in the morning in empty stomach. Note that it is better to avoid fruit after meals.

Take minimum amount of conventional food (rice or chapatti). Try to give up protein or fat rich food and take plenty of vegetables. It is better to take very light diet like *Khoi* in Bengali, at the time of dinner.

By this way one can remain active and energetic by taking more of Bio-energy from green and coloured pigments, instead of taking Chemical-energy from our conventional food. Normally 500 Kcal to 1000 Kcal of bioflavonoid-enriched diet is sufficient to maintain your health without any adverse effect whatsoever. Initially you may feel bit uneasy, but after two or three weeks your stomach size will be reduced to normal and you will not feel unwanted feeling of appetite.

In this process, you will not only loose extra amount of fat steadily, but also you will get rid of many diseases in your life. Above all you will look more attractive and glamorous.

> **BEWARE OF OBESITY! AVOID ACCUMULATION OF FAT BY TAKING PLENTY OF BIO-HERBS WITH BIO-TONE PLUS AND BOOSTER. CHANGE YOUR FOOD-HABIT BY TAKING MORE VEGETABLES.**

*   *   *

DISEASE OF PANCREAS: DIABETES MELLITUS OR BLOOD SUGAR

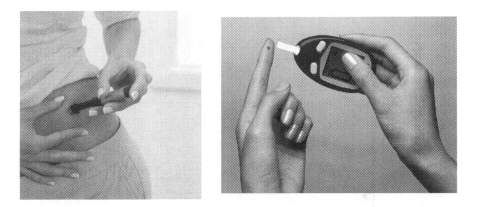

If greed for food cannot be controlled, treatment of diabetes becomes impossible. Diabetes is having genetic taint however, triggered by environmental factors like mental tension and wariness, obesity, overeating, eating of junk-foods containing preservatives, sedentary lifestyle, lack of physical labour, air and water pollution, excessive use of chemical fertilizer and pesticide in agriculture, and perhaps consumption of genetically modified foods. Whatever may be underlying cause, controlled diet with low calorie intake is the main treatment for the patients of diabetes.

Diabetes is the dysfunction of Pancreas (endocrine gland) and insulin hormone. There are two types of diabetes—type 1 or diabetes insidious and type 2 or diabetes mellitus. In type 1 diabetes, pancreas does not produce any insulin (or produce very little quantity). In type 2 diabetes pancreas secrets insulin, but the insulin is not fully utilized due to faulty metabolism. Hence glucose level increases in blood.

Diabetes is a destructive type disease (like cancer) and slowly affects all vital organs like kidney, heart, liver, nervous system (diabetic neuropathy), gum, skin and especially eyes (diabetic retinopathy, diabetic cataract). Unfortunately spread of diabetes in India has become alarming, but there is no effective treatment established till now.

Treatment:

It is mandatory to take Bio-Tone Plus and Booster for treatment of diabetes. Being a destructive disease in nature, one initially needs large doses of these two medicines, depending on the blood-sugar level. For example, one may need 1-3 doses Bio-Tone Plus and 1-2 doses Booster, to be taken twice daily—at the time of breakfast, lunch or dinner (total 6-10 doses daily). Medicines are to be taken at the time of taking food to exhibit the best result.

Along with the medicine, take 1-2 full glasses of juice of coriander leaves (or similar type of green leaves) and coloured fruits in empty stomach twice or thrice daily—in the morning and evening, at least half an hour before taking food. Alternatively take plenty of juice of pumpkin (*Lau* in Bengali or *Lauki* in Hindi or *Dudhi* in Marathi). Certain herbs like *Neem* and *Gulancha* in Bengali also reduce blood sugar to a great extent. Remember, you will not achieve good result without taking high doses of above medicines in combination with juice of green leaves (or coloured fruits) mentioned above.

It is compulsory to take Sugar-Tablet (10-12 tablets daily) after food which moderately reduces blood-sugar level. In addition, patients must take plenty of Bio-Herbs (4-6 spoons daily) for detoxification and providing 'natural vitamins' and 'dietary fiber'. Take Shakti-Raj (1-3 caps daily) for proper digestion and assimilation of nutrients from food. Brush your teeth twice daily by Danta-Raj herbal toothpowder and to supplement magnesium in your body. This will also prevent diabetic cataract and sensitivity of your teeth and gum.

Initially check the blood-sugar level (Fasting and PP) weekly and glycosylated hemoglobin occasionally at 4-6 months interval. Also check your lipid profile once in a year or so. If your results come to satisfactory, you may adjust the dose of medicine depending on the situation. It is worth noting that your allied problems such as protection of vision, skin problem, swelling of gum, arthritic pain, high pressure, high cholesterol, neurological problems, etc. will be under control if our medicines are taken regularly. In this respect, the medicines should be continued for whole life.

The greatest advantage of taking our medicine is that you will never face any problem of hypoglycemia. Medicines will also prevent 'diabetic neuropathy', which is a serious problem of many aged diabetic patients.

Recommended Diet:

Plenty of green chlorophyll and coloured pigments (bioflavonoid) must be taken from fresh green leaves, coloured vegetables, fruits and non-toxic coloured flowers. Avoid nitrogenous food, especially animal protein—this may appear to be contradictory, but the scientific reason is that the protein produces more ammonia, which becomes difficult to excrete from body. Reduce fat intake, instead add more vegetables in your diet. Diabetic patients must chew their food many times to ensure secretion of more saliva for digestion.

If you take sufficient bioflavonoid, your calorie requirement will be reduced to a great extent. Try to avoid rice—instead take chapatti in breakfast and lunch and very light food like *Khoi* in Bengali, at the time of dinner (sometimes taking only *Khoi* with *Musur Dal* soup or *Khatta Dahi* throughout the day proves to be very effective).

Remember, majority of patients, not habituated with insulin therapy, respond quickly with our system of treatment mentioned above. Patients already taking anti-diabetic allopathic medicines should not abruptly stop the medicine—reduce the dose only after having satisfactory blood-test result.

DIABETES MELLITUS	=	START HIGH DOSES OF BIO-TONE PLUS AND BOOSTER DAILY	+	ADDITIONALLY TAKE SUGAR-TABLET (COMPULSORY), SHAKTI-RAJ, BIO-HERB & DANTA-RAJ	+	IT IS COMPULSORY TO TAKE 1-2 GLASSES OF JUICE OF CORIANDER LEAVES OR JUICE OF PUMPKIN OR *GULANCHA* DAILY—IN EMPTY STOMACH, IN THE MORNING

SLOWLY TAPER DOWN THE EXISTING MEDICINES YOU ARE IN USE, DEPENDING ON THE BLOOD-TEST RESULT. DO NOT ABRUPTLY STOP THE ALLOPATHIC MEDICINES, BECAUSE EFFECT OF ABOVE MENTIONED TREATMENT VARIES FROM PATIENT TO PATIENT.

PATIENTS HAVING HIGH BLOOD-SUGAR FOR LONG PERIOD, SAY 10-15 YEARS, SHOULD CONTINUE THIS TREATMENT ALONGWITH REDUCED DOSE OF ALLOPATHIC DRUG. FOR THEM MIXED SYSTEM OF TREATMENT IS BEST AND EFFECTIVE.

> ### IT IS ALMOST COMPULSORY TO TAKE JUICE OF FRESH PUMPKIN AND *GULANCHA* OR 20-40 PIECES GREEN *NEEM* LEAVES IN EMPTY STOMACH BY ALL DIABETIC PATIENTS IRRESPECTIVE OF TAKING OTHER MEDICINES.

*　　*　　*

SIMILARITY OF TREATMENT BETWEEN CANCER AND DIABETES MELLITUS

Cancer and diabetes are characterized by destructive disease—both are generalized disease, affecting all organs of the body. The only difference is destruction in Cancer is rapid whereas in Diabetes, it is slow. Toxins of cancer spread through lymph nodes and glands, whereas in diabetes the blood looses its capacity to utilize insulin (to control glucose), resulting increase of blood-sugar level. Thus the nature of disease is basically same. Therefore it is primary need to focus our attention to correct the metabolic disorder in both the diseases during the treatment.

Bio-Tone Plus and Booster are the main remedy for both cancer and diabetes. Disease being destructive in nature, it is very difficult to select appropriate dose of these two medicines. However dose is to be selected depending on the severity of the disease—thus one may need large doses of Bio-Tone Plus and Booster, say 1-3 doses Bio-Tone Plus and 1-2 doses Booster medicine twice daily (i.e. total 6-10 doses daily), which may be required to be continued for the whole life. Thus the dose or requirement of medicine cannot be compared with respect to other diseases.

In both cases direct detoxification is mandatory by taking plenty of Bio-Herbs daily so that toxins of Cancer or Diabetes expel through stool and urine. By taking green chlorophyll and coloured pigments (bioflavonoid), the adverse effect of toxins reduces to minimum. Juice of certain vegetable and herbs like pumpkin, *gulancha* and *neem* proves to be effective in both cancer and diabetes. Low-protein diet with more vegetables is very much helpful for recovery of the patients.

Thus it is better to adopt integrated system of treatment (i.e. Medicine + Detoxification + intake of Bio-energy) for treatment of cancer and diabetes. In fact treatment of cancer and diabetes is basically same.

* * *

PREVENT CANCER, AIDS AND DREADFUL DISEASES

It has not been possible to establish satisfactory treatment of formidable diseases like Cancer and AIDS or suitable medicines are discovered yet. Therefore, it is better to learn about ways to prevent Cancer, AIDS and other dreadful diseases like Diabetes, Cardiovascular disease or Heart attack.

No disease appears all on a sudden without having any logical background. Diseases are caused by genetic taint, triggered by environmental factors such as pollution (air, water, food and heavy metal), microwave pollution and intake of genetically modified foods. Psychological factors also play a significant role to trigger the genetic taint. Out of all these factors, a part is under our control, whereas balance is beyond our control. Therefore, it is wise to adopt medicinal coverage to subside the metabolic disorder. We have in our system powerful medicine for detoxification of toxins accumulated in our body, thus counterbalancing the adverse effect of pollution in our daily life. In addition to above, Nature has provided the most wonderful medicine—green chlorophyll and coloured pigments (bioflavonoid) to protect ourselves from serious diseases.

Take some doses of Bio-Tone Plus and Booster on regular basis to keep the important organs like heart, liver, kidney, eye and nervous system to function in a better way. Take Sugar-Tablet or Liv-Treat and Shakti-Raj with your food to enhance activity of digestive system. Take Bio-Herbs for direct detoxification and supplementing 'dietary fiber' in your body, lack of which is responsible for disease. Use Danta-Raj and Multi-Care to maintain oral hygiene and strength of your gum.

Apply herbal Eye-Drop to protect eyes from microwave-pollution and air-pollution. Be accustomed with Aqua-Fresh herbal bath for keeping your skin healthy and bacteria-free. Take some amount of Bio-energy (green chlorophyll and coloured pigments), which will keep your mitochondria of body-cells more active. We do not put much stress on exercise from practical point of view—simple breathing exercise for few minutes or walking in open air is enough however, if you can afford to practice running or jogging, it is always better.

Don't worry—simple knowledge of maintenance of health will keep you far away from the dreadful diseases.

*　　*　　*

TREATMENT OF DIGESTIVE SYSTEM (ENDOCRINE GLANDS) ACIDITY, GASTRITIS, WEAK DIGESTION, FATTY LIVER DISEASE

Irregular or over-eating, intake of adulterated or preservative-added food, awakening at night, excessive mental pressure, sedentary lifestyle, food allergy, etc., are the main cause of acidity, gastritis and stomach troubles. Besides, by using cheap variety of chemical-mixed mouth and teeth cleaning materials from childhood, the salivary glands of mouth become less active—as a result functioning of food digestion process comes to be sluggish. Gradually liver becomes weak and various types of disease start developing in the body—gastritis, gout, diabetes, high pressure, high cholesterol, fatty liver disease, etc.

During the process of metabolism, blood or circulatory system supply the vital nutrients to the tissue and lymph takes part in draining out the metabolic waste. Liver is the largest gland in the human body, responsible for controlling the digestive system of the body—the food is ultimately converted to glucose by liver. In contrary to our common belief, the liver plays the main role of digestion (metabolic activity) and not the stomach. The root cause of acidity, gas, weak digestion is due to "weakness of Liver" and treatment should be aimed at improving the function or efficiency of Liver.

TREATMENT OF LIVER (ENDOCRINE GLAND) IS THE BEST SOLUTION FOR CHRONIC STOMACH DISEASE

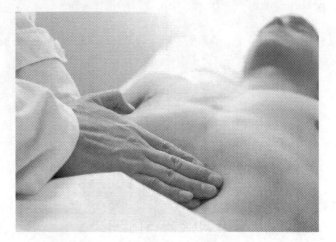

Bio-Tone Plus and Booster are the deep-acting remedies for liver and should be taken for long period to exhibit their action. Initially take 1-2 doses Bio-Tone Plus and 1-2 doses Booster daily for 4-6 months, thereafter take maintenance dose in 2:1 or 1:1 ratio, preferably for the whole life.

Additionally, Sugar-Tablet or Liv-Treat and Shakti-Raj are the effective medicines for treatment of liver. Take Sugar-Tablet or Liv-Treat (8-10 tablets) and 1-3 caps Shakti-Raj along with food (breakfast, lunch or dinner) once or twice daily, as convenient. To supplement 'natural vitamins' and 'dietary fiber' take plenty of Bio-Herbs at bedtime or early in the morning with sufficient water. This will help direct detoxification i.e. expel of toxins from the body through soft stool. Do not take any purgative to remove habitual constipation—Bio-Herbs if taken regularly will slowly remove the tendency of constipation. Brush your teeth twice daily by Danta-Raj herbal toothpowder—this will ensure you bacteria-free mouth and oral hygiene.

Patients of chronic acidity and gas must use Danta-Raj fluoride-free toothpowder for whole life—it is mandatory to keep mouth bacteria-free. It is advised to chew food properly, taking of more vegetable food than non-vegetable stuff. Patients suffering from chronic dysentery will also be benefited from above treatment.

Remember, one-third of your stomach must remain empty during meals. Take less protein (nitrogenous food) and more vegetables to make your diet slightly alkaline. Note that our food habit is inclined towards 'acidic' instead of 'alkaline'—for which we suffer from cluster of diseases.

JAUNDICE AND SPECIAL TREATMENT OF LIVER

The effect of Jaundice or Hepatitis on liver is very serious—it disturbs the liver function. Repeated attack may result change of tissue-structure of liver. The affection on liver may be associated with fever. Under this condition, apply Bio-Tone Plus and Booster daily with multiple doses (say 2-3 doses each Bio-Tone Plus and Booster) at least for 2-3 months.

Depending on the severity of the disease, one may need about half packet each of Bio-Tone Plus and Booster daily. In addition to above repeated doses of 'Fever-Cold' and 'Stomach-Stool' may be beneficial to accelerate the process of cure. Reduce the dose of medicine only after improvement is observed.

Supportive medicine Sugar-Tablet or Liv-Treat, Shakti-Raj, Bio-Herb and Danta-Raj must be taken to get better result.

Patients should take low-protein and low-fat diet and plenty of chlorophyll and coloured pigments (bioflavonoid) from green leaves, coloured vegetables, fruits and non-toxic coloured flowers.

* * *

CONSTIPATION: A COMMON PROBLEM

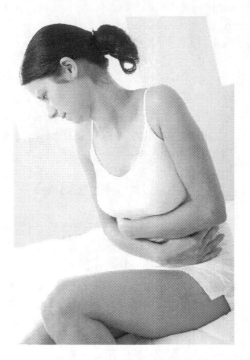

Constipation is a trouble or disease, which seriously disturbs the process of detoxification or expelling toxins from the body. Often constipation is associated with acidity, indigestion, gas, loss of appetite, chronic dysentery, bleeding piles and a number of serious diseases which affect general health of the patient.

Most of the people suffer from inactivity of bowel mainly caused due to lack of peristalsis of the rectum or large intestine due to weakness of nerves. The underlying cause is lack of dietary fiber, chronic diabetes, old age effect, etc.

Bio-Tone Plus and Booster should be taken (say 1 dose each type) daily on long term basis to remove weakness of nerves of the rectum.

Along with the above medicines, take plenty of Bio-Herbs (4-5 spoons daily) daily at bedtime to provide sufficient "dietary fiber" for formation of appropriate type of stool. Drink sufficient water in empty stomach in the morning. Patients having weakness of liver should also take Sugar-Tablet or Liv-Treat and Shakti-Raj on regular basis. Magnesium based Danta-Raj herbal toothpowder has also certain function to eradicate constipation—brush your teeth twice daily. All these medicines will also remove problem of acidity, gas, bleeding piles, etc. and enhance the digestive power of the stomach.

By this way one can get rid of constipation without taking purgatives (like *Sonapata*), which are widely used for movement of bowels.

> **YOU WILL SOON GET RID OF CONSTIPATION BY TAKING PLENTY OF BIO-HERB AT BEDTIME AND DRINKING SUFFICIENT WATER IN THE MORNING IN EMPTY STOMACH.**

TREATMENT OF BLEEDING PILES, FISTULA SURGERY IS NOT THE SOLUTION

The outcome of chronic and prolonged constipation is piles and fistula—patients suffer from ulcer in rectum, blood comes out with stool and sometimes pus oozes out indicating development of fistula.

The existing treatment of Piles or Fistula is very disappointing—often patients are to undergo for surgical operation, sometimes even twice or thrice. The after-effect of surgery is equally disappointing—sometimes the problem of constipation becomes more due to damage of nerves responsible for peristalsis of the rectum.

Bleeding and constipation can be minimized by taking Bio-Tone Plus and Booster continuously on long term basis. Initially take 1-2 doses each Bio-Tone Plus and Booster for 2-3 months, thereafter take maintenance dose in 2:1 or 1:1 ratio. Take plenty of Bio-Herbs at bedtime or in the morning and take sufficient water. Additionally take Sugar-Tablet or Liv-Treat and Shakti-Raj at the time of taking your food. Use Danta-Raj herbal toothpowder twice daily to supplement magnesium in your body. In case of sensation of itching or feeling of rawness on your anus, apply few drops of concentrated lotion Multi-Care or dilute lotion Aqua-Fresh on anus.

Continue the medicines for a year or so—you will be surprised to learn that surgery is not at all required for treatment of Piles and Fistula. It is always better to continue the medicines lifelong, for general maintenance of health.

* * *

TREATMENT OF BLOOD OR CIRCULATORY SYSTEM HIGH CHOLESTEROL, HIGH PRESSURE AND HEART DISEASE

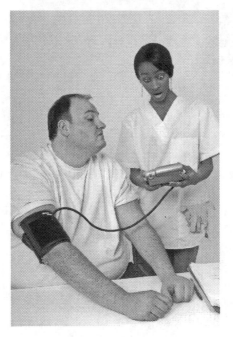

Cardiovascular disease is caused for various reasons such as air pollution, taking adulterated and packed food, genetically modified food-grain, excessive mental pressure, inadequate rest and sleep, less physical labour or exercise, use of excessive oil and spicy food, overeating and so on.

Heart disease is primarily a nerve-related problem. S-A node, A-V node and Bundle of His control the function of heart—any imbalance of these nerves leads to sino-arterial block or atrioventricular block or A-V block at level of bundle branches. Irregularity of pulse (e.g. bradycardia, tachycardia) is also due to faulty signal of nervous system. Thus majority of heart disease is of psychosomatic in origin.

On the other hand liver plays a significant role to determine the composition of blood (plasma-lipoprotein content in blood). In fact liver is responsible for synthesis of HDL, LDL, VLDL, Apo-A, Apo-B, etc.—the imbalance of these lipoproteins is the cause of heart diseases like high pressure, high cholesterol, etc.

Though there are several other causes (like genetic factor) of heart disease, we should mainly focus our attention on improvement of function of nerves and liver, to achieve satisfactory result.

TREATMENT OF CARDIOVASCULAR DISEASE, TONIC FOR HEART

Bio-Tone Plus and Booster are deep-acting remedy to restore harmony between nerve and liver. Initially take 1-2 doses each Bio-Tone Plus and Booster daily for 3-4 months, thereafter take maintenance dose in 2:1 ratio. It is better to continue the medicines for whole life.

Additionally, take 8-10 Sugar-Tablet or Liv-Treat tablets and 1-3 caps Shakti-Raj at the time of lunch or dinner, to improve the function of liver. Take plenty of Bio-Herbs to expel toxins accumulated in the body due to pollution from air, water, food and other external or internal factors. Brush your teeth twice daily by Danta-Raj herbal toothpowder, which will also supplement magnesium in your body.

Take sufficient quantity of chlorophyll and coloured pigments (bioflavonoid) to upgrade the function of lymphatic system or the lymph glands. Green leaves, coloured vegetables, fruits and non-toxic coloured flowers (all in un-cooked condition) are the main source of chlorophyll and bioflavonoid. Make habit of taking 3-4 glasses of juice containing green chlorophyll and coloured pigments. Juice of fresh pumpkin is also very much effective in heart disease. Such juices should always be taken in empty stomach, and not after food. Take more vegetables, low nitrogenous diet (i.e. less protein) and oils. Do not overeat—always keep 1/3rd of your stomach empty. Reduce mental pressure by leading a simple and pious life by keeping faith in Almighty, as far as practicable.

During the treatment check periodically Blood Pressure, Lipid Profile and test for ECG. Checking of Apo-A and Apo-B lipoproteins are also important to assess the possibility of heart attack.

Remember, if you are careful in the beginning, you can easily avoid bypass surgery or fitment of pacemaker in your life!

*   *   *

TREATMENT OF LYMPH-BLOOD DISORDER CHRONIC SKIN DISEASE, ECZEMA, PSORIASIS

The skin disease indicates weak resistant power of immune system of the body. Capability of functioning our kidney and rectum is reduced for various reasons, such as pollution of air, taking adulterated food, less intake of vegetables and effect of diseases like diabetes, constipation, acidity, gas, piles, etc. As a result the poison or toxin stored in our body finds difficulty to come out through urine and stool. So if it continues for long the blood becomes impure due to accumulation of toxins—thus to ensure safety, our natural system tries to expel the surplus amount of toxin through our skin. This is the main cause of skin disease. However, we should never forget the other important cause of skin disease—the deficiency of immunity system of the body which does not provide sufficient resistance to the skin against harmful bacteria or fungus.

Hence it is mandatory to purify the blood and upgrade the immunity system of the body in best possible way, by taking internal medicines.

TREATMENT OF ECZEMA, ITCHING OF SKIN, FALLING OF HAIR

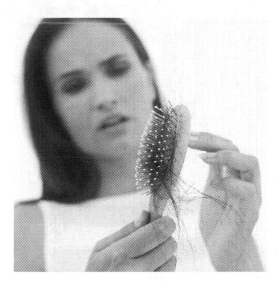

Bio-Tone Plus and Booster are the powerful medicines for all types of skin diseases. These two medicines have capability to purify blood and activate the glands to drain out excess toxins from the body. Take 1-2 doses of Bio-Tone Plus daily and half the quantity Booster on long term basis to get satisfactory result.

Sugar-Tablet or Liv-Treat and Shakti-Raj are also high grade medicines to maintain purity of blood. Take 8-10 Sugar-Tablet or Liv-Treat tablets and 1-3 caps Shakti-Raj daily during food (breakfast, lunch or dinner) on regular basis. Take plenty of Bio-Herbs (4-5 spoons) at bedtime or in the morning to directly expel the toxins accumulated in the blood, by process of detoxification. On the affected area, apply Multi-Care or Aqua-Fresh herbal lotion to subside itching of the skin. Intake of Fever-Cold in repeated doses also helps subsiding itching sensation of the skin.

For hair-fall due to dandruff, herbal bath with Multi-Care or Aqua-Fresh must be taken in addition to internal treatment for purification of blood. Temporarily stop using common soap or shampoo and clean your head with herbal *Ritha*-soaked water. Add plenty of green leaves (chlorophyll), coloured fruits and non-toxic coloured flowers in your daily diet. Remember, hair-fall can be easily prevented with internal medicines and appropriate diet.

TREATMENT OF PSORIASIS OF COMPLICATED TYPE

It is not difficult to cure Psoriasis in our system of treatment. Take 1-2 doses each Bio-Tone Plus and Booster daily on regular basis—the deep acting drugs for all types of skin disease. Continue the medicines at least for 1 or 2 years.

Detoxify the accumulated toxins of your blood directly by Bio-Herb, to be taken plenty (4-5 spoons) at bedtime or in the morning. Take sufficient water in empty stomach in the morning. Toxins will come out of your body through soft stool and the blood will be thus purified. In addition take Sugar-Tablet or Liv-Treat and Shakti-Raj in combination regularly, to be taken twice daily during food. Apply Multi-Care herbal lotion on the affected area of the skin to subside sensation of itching.

For patients of Psoriasis, it is mandatory to take sufficient amount of green chlorophyll and coloured pigments (bioflavonoid), available from green leaves, coloured vegetables, fruits and non-toxic coloured flowers. Regular intake of 15-20 pieces fresh green *neem* leaves and raw-garlic in empty stomach in the morning proves to be beneficial for the patients.

Remember, Psoriasis can be cured easily with medicines and appropriate diet.

> **TOXINS MUST BE REMOVED EVERYDAY FROM YOUR BODY TO ACHIEVE SMOOTH CURE DURING TREATMENT OF SKIN DISEASE. ALWAYS APPLY MULTI-CARE HERBAL LOTION TO SUBSIDE THE ITCHING PROBLEM.**

*   *   *

TREATMENT OF

DISEASES OF RESPIRATORY SYSTEM

Lung play vital role in supplying oxygen to the blood through numerous aperture called alveoli. Exchange of oxygen and carbon dioxide (waste product of blood) takes place through numerous blood-carrying capillary vessels of the lung. Function of oxygen is to supply energy to our tissue and nervous system, deficiency of which may even threaten our life.

Underlying cause of disorder of respiratory system such as cold and cough, infection of lung, bronchitis, pneumonia, etc. is nothing but the deficiency of the immune system of the body. Children, who are yet to develop sufficient immune cells or immunoglobulin due to hypo-activity of lymphatic system, generally suffer more on respiratory trouble such as chronic cold and cough. On the other hand old people also suffer from chronic respiratory problem mainly due to prolonged use of various types of drugs in their life. In fact response of the common drugs in old age becomes slow due to obvious reasons.

It is therefore essential to treat children and old people more effectively to cut short their sufferings. Bio-Tone Plus and Booster are the main medicines for application in all diseases related to the respiratory system.

CHRONIC COLD AND COUGH, CHRONIC AND ACUTE BRONCHITIS, PNEUMONIA

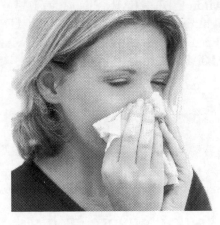

Depending on the severity, initially take Bio-Tone Plus and Booster in large doses for 2-3 days. Take these two medicines repeatedly—you may need 4-5 doses of each type of medicine daily to overcome the problem. After the acute phase is over or feeling of rawness of your chest or throat goes away, take maintenance dose of these two medicines (say 1-3 doses Bio-Tone Plus and 1 dose Booster) for few days. Incase of spasmodic cough due to throat infection, which is more of nervous origin, frequent doses of Fever-Cold or few drops Multi-Care may exhibit good result to subside the irritation within a short time.

For old people, it is better to continue 1-2 doses Bio-Tone Plus daily and one-third the quantity Booster on regular basis for the whole life to keep their nervous system active, along with the protection of lung from infection, cough and phlegm.

Smokers need not be worried on bad effect of smoking—regular use of Bio-Tone Plus and Booster will keep your lung clear. Take 1-2 doses Bio-Tone Plus daily and half the quantity Booster regularly—medicines will help lung to expel slowly the accumulated phlegm and will never allow drying up the cough which may lead to formation of bronchitis.

Remember, Bio-Tone Plus is the wonderful medicine for all types of respiratory or lung problem. Take repeatedly when you are in crisis.

It is interesting to note that taking frequent bath in cold water during bronchitis with high fever elevates the immunity potential against cold and cough. In this process additionally take multiple doses of Bio-Tone Plus and Booster for better result.

PULMONARY DISEASE

IN INDUSTRIAL AND URBAN AREA

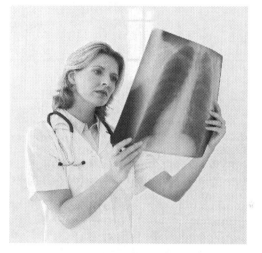

People in industrial area, residing at the vicinity of coal mines or stone-crushing factories are subjected to serious pollution from dust or silicon. As a result, their alveoli get closed in many places of the lung which may lead to feeling of suffocation. Sometimes they become sufferer of chronic cold and cough, which becomes difficult to cure.

People residing in urban area also suffer from air pollution, ranging from mild to high grade—many of them suffer from cold and cough throughout the year, especially during the change of weather. This is particularly marked for old people—generally they face difficulty to expel the phlegm due to sluggishness of nerves.

Bio-Tone Plus and Booster are the medicines to eradicate all respiratory problems. Select the dose of medicine as per the severity of the problem; say 1-3 doses Bio-Tone Plus daily and one-third the quantity Booster. However, it is better to continue the maintenance dose of medicine for whole life.

Breathing exercise (short and long breathing) is always helpful to open up the alveoli of the lung. Certain foods like *Gur* and Honey also help to function as expectorant or cleansing agent of lung, if taken regularly.

ASTHMA, BRONCHIAL ASTHMA

The main cause of asthma is prolonged sufferings from cough and cold, susceptibility to catch cold, intake of adulterated food, allergy from dust, etc. People residing in urban area or industrial belt are subjected to high-grade of air pollution, often toxic gases like ammonia, sulpher dioxide, carbon monoxide and especially fine dust of silicon or carbon. Persons sensitive to air pollution, are generally become victim of asthma.

The underlying cause of asthma is lack of immunity of the body against specific allergen showing malfunction of antigen-antibody defense mechanism. Lymphatic nodes and glands play vital role in immunity system of the body by producing immunoglobulin through a signal-communication network of the brain i.e. nervous system. Blood or circulatory system is the carrier of the lymphocyte cells, producing immunoglobulin or immunity mechanism.

Bio-Tone Plus and Booster are high-grade remedy for treatment of asthma. Depending on the severity or frequency of attack, take regularly Bio-Tone Plus and Booster, say 1-3 doses Bio-Tone Plus and one-third the quantity Booster daily, and continue the medicines over a long period, preferably for lifelong.

By this way immunity against dust and cold will be developed slowly to resist the asthmatic attack. Sometimes it is beneficial to take repeated dose of Fever-Cold during attack of asthma. Additionally take General medicines (Sugar-Tablet or Liv-Treat, Shakti-Raj, Bio-Herb and Danta-Raj) to accelerate the process of cure. Asthmatic patients should take sufficient green chlorophyll and coloured pigments (bioflavonoid) to develop more immunity of their body.

If necessary, use inhaler on SOS basis. If our medicines are continued for about 1 or 2 years, gradually the necessity of taking inhaler gets reduced.

APPLY BIO-TONE PLUS AND BOOSTER BLINDLY ON ANY TYPE OF LUNG-RELATED DISEASE

* * *

TREATMENT OF ARTHRITIS, JOINT PAIN, GOUT, FROZEN SHOULDER

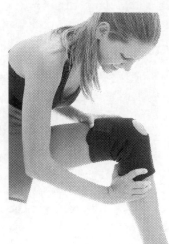

Taking of adulterated food, incomplete treatment after bone injury, long use of fluoride-mixed tooth-cleaning items from childhood, weakness of liver and digestive system, chronic constipation, problem of acidity and gas, wastage of bone-calcium during menopause, etc. are the root causes of arthritis and joint pain. Arthritis is a sort of metabolic disorder—prolonged use of pain-relieving medicines sometimes makes the case more complicated.

Treatment:

Bio-Tone Plus and Booster are the high-graded medicines for all types of arthritis. Initially take 1-3 doses each Bio-Tone Plus and Booster daily for 2-3 months, thereafter take maintenance dose in 2:1 or 1:1 ratio. These medicines will take care of joint pain and rigidity of muscle. Aged persons generally suffer from multiple problems—for them it is always better to continue these two medicines for whole life.

Besides, to clean blood and protection against gout resulting from high uric acid, take Shakti-Raj and Sugar-Tablet or Liv-Treat for the whole life. Apply Multi-Care lotion on the painful area. For constipation and rapid detoxification of toxins from the body, take plenty of Bio-Herb 1 or 2 at bedtime and drink sufficient water in the morning in empty stomach to expel toxins from body through soft stool. Females will get sufficient nutrition of muscles and bones from above medicines, which will prevent them from osteoporosis during their menopausal period. Patients of arthritis must use fluoride-free Danta-Raj herbal toothpowder twice daily for whole life—it is also essential to make mouth bacteria-free.

Patients of arthritis should reduce their protein intake because amino-acids in excess lead to increase of ammonia level which is toxic in nature. Therefore, it is better if they consume more vegetables than protein-rich diet. Vegetable-enriched diet and Sugar-Tablet or Liv-Treat will make the diet alkaline (note that one of the major cause of arthritis is we take more acidic food than of alkaline food). Intake of green chlorophyll and coloured pigments (bioflavonoid) available from green leaves, vegetables, fruits and non-toxic coloured flowers will greatly reduce arthritic taint. Additionally take raw-garlic and 15-20 pieces fresh green *neem* leaves in empty stomach as preventive measure of arthritis.

In case of injury, X-Ray is suggested first to check if there is any fracture or hair-line crack. Take repeated doses of Bio-Tone Plus & Booster and apply Multi-Care lotion on the injured area. Additionally you may have to consult orthopedic doctor as per requirement.

Remember, initial stage of arthritis can be cured very easily. Aged patients suffering from high-grade arthritis or osteoarthritis cannot be fully cured by any system of treatment—however, medicines will help to control the problem. In addition to intake of medicines, Physiotherapy or Electrotherapy is recommended for faster relief from pain.

> **RAPID DETOXIFICATION IS NECESSARY TO SUBSIDE PAIN OF ARTHRITIS AND GOUT. TAKE PLENTY OF BIO-HERBS FOR DIRECT EXPELLING OF TOXINS FROM THE BODY THROUGH SOFT STOOL. ADDITIONALLY TAKE BIO-TONE PLUS AND BOOSTER ON REGULAR BASIS FOR INDIRECT DETOXIFICATION. SHAKTI-RAJ, SUGAR-TABLET OR LIV-TREAT AND DANTA-RAJ ARE EFFECTIVE MEDICINES FOR LONG TERM TREATMENT.**

> **FOR ACUTE OR CHRONIC CASES OF ARTHRITIS, IT IS BETTER TO UNDERGO PHYSIOTHERAPY TREATMENT ALONG WITH TREATMENT BY MEDICINE TO GET FASTER RELIEF.**

*   *   *

TREATMENT OF ARSENIC POISONING

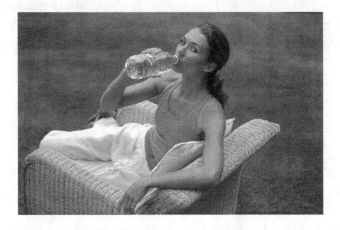

Main source of arsenic poisoning is shallow tubewell water. Due to extensive use of underground water for agriculture and irrigation in our country, the water-level gradually goes down—as a result, concentration of arsenic in water increases. When the percentage of arsenic in water crosses tolerable limit, the water is said to be poisonous for human use. Similarly, in big cities, large amount of water is pumped out from underground for drinking purpose. Thus the groundwater level goes down and we face arsenic poisoning.

Arsenic poisoning is characterized by intolerable itching, appearance of round spot like ring-worm on the skin, etc. Many people are affected with skin-cancer and may even loose their lives.

Treatment:

If itching is noticed on the body, apply Sonali antiseptic cream or Multi-Care herbal lotion immediately on the affected area of the skin—the itching will be subsided within a few days. Take repeatedly Bio-Tone Plus and Booster in combination as internal medicine for treatment of arsenic poisoning. In addition to above, take Fever-Cold frequently, even at 5 to 10 minutes interval to make subside the violent itching on the skin. Take Aqua-Fresh herbal bath for external protection of skin.

Take plenty of Bio-Herb (Nos. 1 or 2) for detoxification of toxins resulting from arsenic poisoning. Herbs must be taken in large doses (5-6 spoons daily) to expel the accumulated toxin from the body through loose motion. It is better to take Shakti-Raj tonic and Sugar-Tablet or Liv-Treat, in addition to above medicines.

Take necessary preventive measures to arrest the effect of arsenic poisoning by taking 1-2 doses Bio-Tone Plus daily and half the quantity Booster on regular basis—these are the best preventive medicine of arsenic poisoning.

The condition of patient further improves if sufficient green chlorophyll and coloured pigments (bioflavonoid) are taken daily on regular basis.

ARSENIC POISONING IS THE ROOT CAUSE OF MANY SKIN DISEASES. PREVENTIVE MEDICINES ARE BIO-TONE PLUS, BOOSTER AND BIO-HERBS.

---

* * *

TREATMENT OF FLUORIDE POISONING

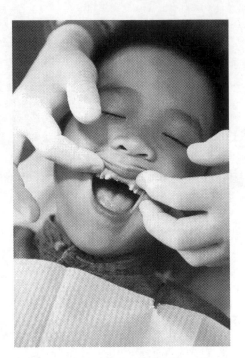

The fluoride poisoning, like arsenic poisoning, is seen in various regions of Asia, particularly in India. A little quantity of fluoride is always present in water. Besides, cheap varieties of tooth-cleaning items are the main sources of fluoride contamination. Everybody knows that fluorine is the most reactive element—it rapidly makes reaction with Calcium present in bones. Erosion takes place in bones, especially in the joints—as a result density of bone decreases and thus creates osteoporosis disease. In fact the underlying cause of all types of erosion of bones such as arthritis, osteoarthritis, waist-pain, spondylitis, slip-disk, decaying of tooth, etc. are the direct or indirect effect of Fluoride poisoning.

Treatment:

Specific treatment of fluoride poisoning is not known. But for preventive treatment, non-fluoride herbal toothpowder Danta-Raj must be used for the whole life. Take 2-3 doses Bio-Tone Plus daily and half the quantity Booster to combat with fluoride poisoning. These two medicines are very effective to reduce pain of bones, especially the joints and maintenance dose should be continued for whole life. Take plenty of Bio-Herb (No. 1 or 2) at bedtime and drink sufficient water in the morning in empty stomach to expel accumulated toxins from body through soft stool.

Additionally take Sugar-Tablet or Liv-Treat and Shakti-Raj to improve general condition of the patient. Green chlorophyll and coloured pigments (bioflavonoid) should be taken in sufficient quantity to achieve better result.

To reduce the pain, apply Multi-Care pain-relieving herbal lotion on the affected area of the bone. Intake of Fever-Cold medicine repeatedly, sometimes gives relief from pain.

FLUORIDE POISONING IS THE MAJOR CAUSE OF ARTHRITIS AND BONE-DISEASE. PREVENTIVE MEDICINES ARE BIO-TONE PLUS, BOOSTER AND BIO-HERBS.

---

*   *   *

TREATMENT OF OLD AGE PROBLEMS (GERIATRIC DISEASE)

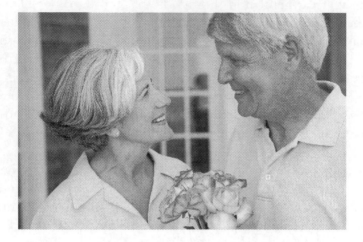

Most of the old people suffer from three major problems—disease of respiratory system like persistent cold and cough, pneumonia, etc., disease of nervous system like general weakness, forgetfulness, or shortage of memory, Parkinson's disease and disease of digestive system such as indigestion, acidity and gas. All these problems are part and parcel of the old age, especially the persistent cold and cough, which becomes difficult to cure in old age.

Don't worry—there may be hundreds of problems in old age, but we especially look into the protection of nerves, glands and vital organs of the body—thus minimizing your problems at the old age. Take 1-2 doses Bio-Tone Plus daily and one-third the quantity Booster in the old age to minimize the old-age problems. Take Sugar-Tablet or Liv-Treat and Shakti-Raj at the time of food to reduce the stomach problems. Take plenty of Bio-Herbs containing 'natural vitamins' and 'dietary fiber' and drink sufficient water to get rid of old-age constipation. Use Danta-Raj twice daily to supplement magnesium and ensuring bacteria-free mouth.

Minimize your intake of food, especially protein—instead take more carbohydrate, vegetables and fruits. Green chlorophyll and coloured pigments (bioflavonoid) will enhance your life force to a great extent.

Remember, disease cannot be totally avoided in old age, but can be controlled easily by using regularly the above medicines for 'metabolic disorder'.

> **TAKE BIO-TONE PLUS AND BOOSTER REGULARLY IN 3:1 RATIO FROM 50 YEARS OF AGE AND REMAIN PRACTICALLY DISEASE-FREE FOR REST OF YOUR LIFE.**

* * *

TREATMENT OF CHILDREN'S DISEASES (PEDIATRIC DISEASES)

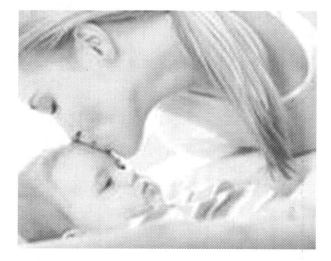

Diagnosis of disease of children is comparatively difficult because they cannot express their problems to the doctors. Especially infants and babies who have not yet learned to speak require elaborate checking by doctors to find out the problem—therefore, there is every possibility of incorrect diagnosis. Moreover, we find difficulty to find out the appropriate medicine as well as the dose of the remedy.

In our system, selection of medicine and treatment of disease is very simple. In fact the medicines which are applicable to the adult are also applicable to the little children. The medicines are non-toxic in all respect; hence you need not be worried about dose, because large doses of medicine will not be harmful to your children. Apply the medicines from your experience on your children.

Bio-Tone Plus and Booster are the leading medicines for all types of fever, cold, cough, tonsillitis, pharengitis, skin disease and so on. Depending on the severity, apply the medicines repeatedly (say 2-3 doses each type) to achieve cure in shortest time. These two medicines will also boost up defense mechanism of your children to a great extent. If you do not have these medicines with you, apply at least 'Fever-Cold' liquid medicine, which will also work efficiently to do away the problems of your child.

Children generally have tendency to suffer from sudden diarrhea or dysentery or constipation or problem of gas in abdomen. Apply Stomach-Stool medicine repeatedly in crisis. Sometimes little babies get fever from stomach trouble which is difficult to detect—in this case apply both Fever-Cold and Stomach-Stool blindly to achieve cure in a short time.

Children often get injured (blow or bleeding) while playing with their friends. Don't worry—apply Multi-Care pain-relieving and antiseptic lotion or Sonali herbal antiseptic cream, whichever you have in your stock. In case of bleeding from cuts or wounds, apply the same lotion or cream and give Fever-Cold or Bio-Tone Plus or Booster as internal medicine.

Thus majority of your problems will be easily resolved by applying the simple and limited number of medicines. You need not wait for diagnosis or the result of pathological test—simply apply the medicines during onset of the problem.

BIO-TONE PLUS AND BOOSTER, IF TAKEN REGULARLY,
WILL UPGRADE IMMUNITY SYSTEM OF YOUR
CHILD TO A GREAT EXTENT. YOUR CHILD WILL BE
PRACTICALLY FREE FROM COMMON DISEASE.

*   *   *

TREATMENT OF FEMALE DISEASES
(GYNECOLOGICAL PROBLEMS)

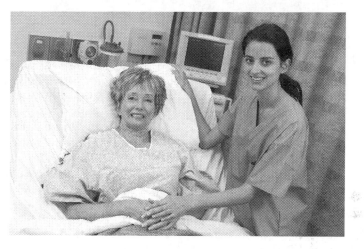

During puberty, majority of our little sisters suffer from painful menstruation (dysmenorrhoea) and do not visit doctors due to their shyness. On the other hand, our aged mothers suffer from array of problems during their menopause—many of them suffer from leucorrhoea, excessive bleeding (menorrohgia), irregular menstruation, flashing sensation at different parts of the body and osteoporosis due to wastage of calcium of the body. Nowadays diseases like tumour or polyp in uterus or swelling of lymph node of the breast have become so common that many of them have to undergo surgical treatment, because they cannot avail suitable treatment in time, due to many reasons.

It is interesting to note that all female diseases are due to malfunction of lymphatic system—lymphatic nodes, endocrine and exocrine glands play vital role. Thus it is better to treat the glands instead of applying medicines for the specific disease.

Bio-Tone Plus and Booster are the deep-acting medicines for all types of gynecological disorders. Initially take 1-2 doses each Bio-Tone Plus and Booster daily for 2-3 months, thereafter take maintenance dose in 2:1 or 1:1 ratio. Medicines should be taken for a year or so to overcome the problem. Aged women having many other problems should continue the medicines for whole life. Additionally take plenty of Bio-Herbs to detoxify and to provide "natural vitamins" and "dietary fiber" in your body. Remember, Bio-Herbs are extremely useful to prevent osteoporosis and tumours of glands such as tumours of uterus or breasts. Take 1-3 caps Shakti-Raj regularly to prevent cancerous tendency on any part of your body. Take 5-6 Sugar-Tablet or Liv-Treat tablets for digestive problems and use Danta-Raj herbal toothpowder to supplement magnesium in your body.

Thus treatment of gynecological disorders is much simplified in our system of medicine—the disease may be anything, but the medicines are same.

> **BIO-TONE PLUS, BOOSTER AND BIO-HERBS ARE THE HIGH-GRADE PREVENTIVE MEDICINES FOR ALL TYPES OF GYNECOLOGICAL PROBLEMS**

* * *

TREATMENT OF SIMPLE AND UNKNOWN TYPE OF FEVER

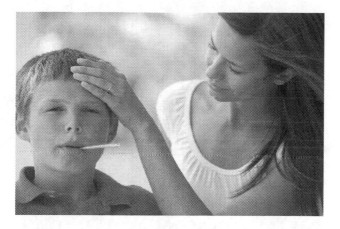

Fever is the outcome of internal ailment characterized by rise of temperature of the body. It is generally caused due to attack of infective virus, bacteria or parasites. As a result we suffer from common flue, tonsillitis, pharengitis, bronchitis, pneumonia, malaria, typhoid, kala-azar, etc. The pathogens react with defense mechanism of the body; thereby toxin is released within the body. In other words fever is caused due to deficiency of the immunity system of the body. Lymphatic nodes play vital role in our defensive mechanism by producing lymphocytes, which in turn produce antibodies or immunoglobulin and protect the body from antigen.

Bio-Tone Plus and Booster act on glands (lymphatic nodes) to improve the defensive mechanism of the body. Depending on the severity of the disease, take repeatedly both the medicines, thus one may require initially 5-6 doses each type of the medicines on the very first day to control the situation.

The main advantage of the application of Bio-Tone Plus and Booster is that the medicines can be applied repeatedly at the time of onset of the disease without running around for pathological tests to identify the type of virus, bacteria or parasite. Thus the fever may be malaria, typhoid, kala-azar, arthritic fever or even any unknown type of fever. If the medicine is applied repeatedly in the beginning, recovery is expected within one or two days. Once the crisis period is over, take maintenance dose of above two medicines. In case you have limited stock of Bio-Tone Plus or Booster, apply 'Fever-Cold' medicine along with the above medicines.

Thus the treatment of fever is much simplified with application of Bio-Tone Plus and Booster.

* * *

CRISIS MANAGEMENT AND TREATMENT AT HOME

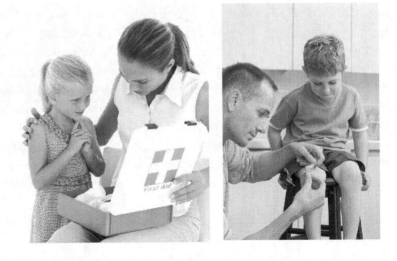

If the disease is not surgical, treatment in most of the cases is simple in our system—take the medicines blindly without scratching your head. For convenience and ready reference, note the following applications of medicines in acute conditions:

High Fever, Fever of unknown type, Flue, Swelling of Glands, Severe Throat Pain:

Take Bio-Tone Plus and Booster repeatedly—you may have to consume 1 packet each on the very first day. Take maintenance dose after the crisis stage is over.

Severe Diarrhea, Watery Stool with or without Vomiting:

Take 5-6 full droppers Multi-Care and 8-10 caps Shakti-Raj in a glass of water and mix the medicines. Stir well and take the medicine in 4-5 doses at an interval of 5-10 minutes. Repeat the medicine till the problem subsides. Alternatively take repeated doses of "Stomach-Stool" say at 5-10 minutes interval.

Bleeding due to Cuts from Sharp Instrument or Knife:

Apply Multi-Care antiseptic, antibacterial and antifungal herbal lotion. Alternatively apply Sonali antiseptic herbal cream to stop bleeding. Bandage the affected area if there is excessive bleeding. To eradicate the possibility of getting tetanus, take Bio-Tone Plus or Booster or Fever-Cold 4-5 times in a day and continue the medicine for a week. Both Multi-Care and Sonali are excellent medicines for quick-healing of wounds after surgical operations.

Blow or Injury on Head, Severe Headache, Migraine, Vertigo:

For all types of head-related problems, take few doses of Bio-Tone Plus and Booster (say 4-6 doses of each type) at 10-15 minutes interval. After the crisis period is over, take maintenance dose.

Burns and Bites of Poisonous Insects such as Bees, Wasps:

Apply Sonali antiseptic cream on affected area. Alternatively apply Multi-Care antiseptic lotion. If possible, take Fever-Cold liquid repeatedly at 5-10 minutes interval.

Urticaria, Ring-like Swelling on Skin, Intolerable Itching of Skin:

Apply Multi-Care antiseptic lotion or Sonali antiseptic cream on the affected area to subside the itching sensation. In all cases it is better to take 4-5 doses each Bio-Tone Plus and Booster. Repeated intake of Fever-Cold liquid medicine will also help.

Painful Swelling of Gum, Toothache, Bleeding of Gum:

Apply Multi-Care antiseptic lotion at least 5-6 times in a day on the painful area. Brush with Danta-Raj herbal toothpowder twice or thrice daily. Take 4-5 doses of Bio-Tone Plus to subside the pain in shortest time.

Severe Bleeding of Piles, Fistula, Blood Dysentery:

Take 8-10 Sugar-Tablet or Liv-Treat tablets 2-3 times in a day. Few doses of Bio-Tone Plus and Booster (say 3-4 doses each type) will be very much helpful to stop bleeding and reduce pain. Repeated dose of Stomach-Stool liquid is also helpful. For chronic constipation take plenty of Bio-Herbs and drink sufficient water in empty stomach. For fistula take Bio-Tone Plus and Booster on regular basis. For itching sensation of anus apply Multi-Care antiseptic lotion. Shakti-Raj also proves to be beneficial in bleeding of piles.

Conjunctivitis, Pain, Rawness of Eye, Sensitive to light:

Apply herbal Eye-Drop few times at 5-10 minutes interval. In addition to above internal medicine Bio-Tone Plus and Booster (say 2-3 doses each type for few days) is also very much helpful to get relief from crisis. Alternatively mix 10-15 drops Multi-Care or 3-4 droppers Aqua-Fresh lotion in a glass or cup of water and wash your eyes; you will get the same result of eye-drop. Direct application of 1 or 2 drops Multi-Care or Aqua-Fresh on eyes is also recommended as a good alternative to eye-drop.

Severe or Shooting Pain anywhere in the body:

Remember Bio-Tone Plus for all types of serious pain (non-surgery type) related to nerve or head—it may be migraine, headache, flashing sensation of nerve, shooting or pulsating pain anywhere in the body. Take repeated doses of Bio-Tone Plus; say at 15-20 minutes interval. You will be surprised to get relief from severe nerve-pain within a short time.

KEEP ALL THE STANDARD MEDICINES IN YOUR HOME-STOCK TO GET IMMEDIATE RESPONSE DURING EMERGENCY.

KEEP ESPECIALLY FEW PACKETS BIO-TONE PLUS, BOOSTER AND A PHIAL OF MULTI-CARE LOTION TO OVERCOME CRISIS OF MANY TYPES.

---

*　*　*

TREATMENT OF PATIENTS SUFFERING FROM ARRAY OF MULTIPLE OR COMPLEX DISEASES

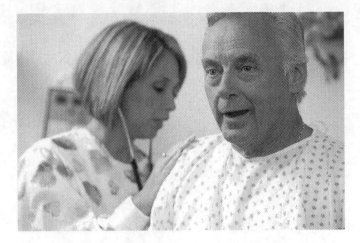

After the age of 35-40 years, we generally find patients are suffering from multiple diseases. These patients at their earlier age, might have suffered from one or two diseases, but time comes when they become victim of a group of chronic diseases such as acidity, indigestion, gas, fatty liver disease, arthritis, high uric acid, high blood pressure, high cholesterol, hypo or hyper thyroidism, chronic cold and cough, skin disease, neurological problems and so on. If the patient is female, she might have additionally developed pre-menopausal or post-menopausal problems such as erratic sensation of flashing of nerves, abdominal pain due to excessive or scanty bleeding, leucorrhoea, tumour on uterus, etc. Also there is a high chance of getting osteoporosis due to excessive loss of calcium during menopause.

How to treat these type of patients, who are suffering from multiple or array of diseases? As per the prevailing practice, the patients are generally treated in accordance with symptom or the disease. But in our system of treatment, patients need not take in account the symptoms or problems. The reason behind our treatment is based on correction of "metabolic disorder" only. You need not therefore, think of individual problem—consider the body as a whole unit and apply the medicines.

Don't worry—blindly apply the remedy for "metabolic disorder" for treatment of multiple diseases. Take Bio-Tone Plus and Booster as principal medicines of nerve, lymph and blood. Depending on the severity, take 2-3 doses Bio-Tone Plus and half or one-third quantity Booster medicine continuously for few months or year. Additionally take General medicines for "metabolic disorder" i.e. Sugar-Tablet or Liv-Treat, Shakti-Raj, Bio-Herb, Danta-Raj, Multi-Care, Aqua-Fresh and Herbal Eye-Drop.

Within a short time (say 3-4 months) you will observe remarkable improvement to all your problems. Thus with a limited number of medicines you can get rid of your multiple problems in shortest period of time. You will be surprised to learn that you have achieved smooth cure without any trouble of visiting at our clinic.

Thus the simple and easy method of cure should be followed as far as practicable.

List of medicines used for treatment of multiple or complex diseases:

Sl. No.	Medicine with reason of application		Special Benefit
1)	**Compulsory medicines for nerve, gland and blood:** Bio-Tone Plus and Booster (use both the medicines)	:	Medicine will take care of nerve, lymph and blood (acts on nerves, glands and all organs of the body). These two medicines will cover about 60% of the whole problems—essential remedies to overcome the crisis. Refer Table-I for evaluation.

2)	**Medicines for better assimilation of food and nutrients:** Sugar-Tablet or Liv-Treat and Shakti-Raj	:	Action of Sugar-Tablet or Liv-Treat is on digestive system and liver. Shakti-Raj acts on blood and digestive system. High importance should be given to correct liver-function.
3)	**Medicines for Detoxification and supplementing Dietary fiber:** Bio-Herb (Nos. 1 & 2)	:	Excellent medicine for direct detoxification. Provides natural vitamins and dietary fibers. Accumulation of toxin in body and lack of dietary fiber are the root cause of disease.
4)	**Medicines for bacteria-free mouth, Skin-care and Eye-care:** Danta-Raj herbal toothpowder and herbal Eye-Drop	:	Danta-Raj and Multi-Care are for bacteria-free mouth and teeth, essential for minimizing stomach problems. Aqua-Fresh is for skin-care, protects from skin disease. Eye-Drop is to protect eye from external pollution (dust and microwaves).
5)	**Bioflavonoid:** Green chlorophyll and coloured pigments of the Nature	:	Always shows great improvement in complex type of diseases. Take plenty of green leaves and coloured fruits or non-toxic coloured flowers in un-cooked condition, especially in cancer, diabetes and cardiovascular disease.

BIO-TONE PLUS AND BOOSTER COVERS 60% OF TOTAL MEDICATION VALUE, REFER TABLE-I. NOTE THAT AGED PEOPLE NEED MORE MEDICINE THAN YOUNGSTER DUE TO AGE-FACTOR.

KEYWORD OF HEALTH	–	• MEDICINE, DIET AND EXERCISE (BIOPATHY SYSTEM OF TREATMENT) • MEDICINE FOR NERVES, GLANDS AND VITAL ORGANS (BIO-TONE PLUS AND BOOSTER) • MEDICINE FOR DIGESTIVE SYSTEM OR LIVER (SUGAR-TABLET OR LIV-TREAT AND SHAKTI-RAJ) • MEDICINE FOR DIRECT DETOXIFICATION (BIO-HERB NOS. 1 & 2) • BACTERIA-FREE MOUTH AND TEETH (DANTA-RAJ AND MULTI-PLUS) • SKIN CARE (AQUA-FRESH) AND EYE CARE (HERBAL EYE-DROP) • NATURAL MEDICINES (GREEN CHLOROPHYLL AND COLOURED PIGMENTS)

*   *   *

ROLE OF SURGERY IN TREATMENT OF CERTAIN DISEASES

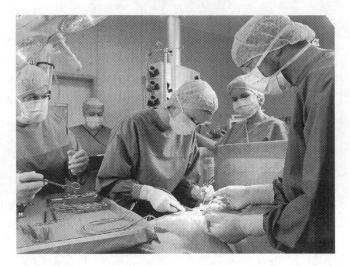

Most of the people have wrong idea that surgery is not a part of Ayurvedic system of medicine. Almost all of us think that we do not advocate or acknowledge the importance of surgery as a part of treatment in Ayurveda. This type of wrong idea has been promulgated amongst us perhaps because the surgery is conducted by allopath doctors only mainly in hospitals where non-surgical treatments are also conducted by allopath doctors.

Going insight about surgery, one must keep in mind that surgery was introduced for the first time in the world by *Charak* and *Sushruta* through Ayurveda system of medicine. Gradually the instruments and methodology of surgery have been upgraded from time to time. In ancient time primitive instruments were in use, whereas in 21st century computerized operation with robotics has been introduced. The advancement of surgery has been made possible due to dedicated research by many scientists and engineers working throughout the world. In fact surgery is a group-activity of scientists, engineers and doctors—it is altogether a different approach or system of treatment, it comes neither in homeopathy, nor in ayurveda or allopathic system of medicine.

Surgery is therefore, altogether a different subject, originally founded by *Charak* and *Sushruta*, which has got no relation with medicinal cure—though we have wrong idea that it is a part of allopathic system. The fact is that surgery is a common subject for all branches of medicines; it may be homeopathy, allopathic or ayurveda. Therefore, our traditional thoughts should be amended accordingly.

The purpose of separating surgery from various systems of medicine is that many homeopaths and ayurvedic doctors do not put any importance on surgery, though introduced by *Charak* and *Sushruta*. One must understand that when there is permanent deformation or massive change of tissue structure, the treatment goes beyond the scope of medicine and no treatment under medicine can bring back the changes to normal. For example, a large lump or a gallstone of comparatively big in size cannot be treated by medicine because such type of change of structure is irreversible type. Homeopathy and ayurveda doctors should advice these cases for surgical operation by referring to the allopathic surgeons or advising for hospitalization, instead of doing futile exercise to cure by medicine. In fact the primary duty of doctors is to judge whether the case is surgical or can be treated by medicine and treat the patients accordingly. We are extremely grateful to those allopathic surgeons, specialist doctors, scientists and especially high-tech engineers who developed modern surgical instruments and medicines, introduced robotics and computers, without which the treatment would have been incomplete.

Remember, surgery is the common platform where all the systems of medicines meet—it may be homeopathy, allopathy or ayurveda. In case of doubt, try first with medicine—if cure is not achieved, refer to the surgeon. Therefore, homeopathy and ayurveda doctors should come closer to surgical treatments and pathological or laboratory tests including advanced tests like USG, CT Scan or MRI. Don't hesitate to avail the benefit of modern surgery—the system which was originally founded by *Charak* and *Sushruta!*

> ## AVAIL BENEFITS OF MODERN SURGERY—THE SUBJECT ORIGINALLY INTRODUCED BY *CHARAK* AND *SUSHRUTA!* DOCTOR'S PRIMARY DUTY IS "IDENTIFICATION" OF THE SURGICAL CASES.

*   *   *

IMPORTANCE OF PATHOLOGICAL OR LABORATORY TEST

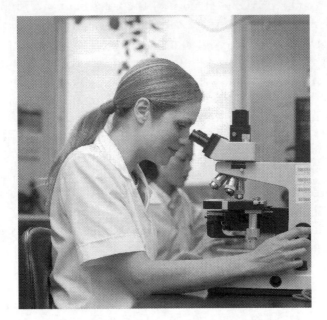

Though we have not elaborated any pathological or laboratory tests, it should not be misinterpreted that we are not in favour of doing any test to diagnose the nature of disease. In fact where necessary, patients must undergo pathological tests. For example, a patient of skin disease will not respond well if he or she is diabetic or having Blood sugar. Therefore, in this case it is mandatory to test for blood sugar and the patient must take medicine in accordance with the treatment of diabetes. Similarly a patient of cardiovascular disease must undergo tests for lipid profile and ECG without which the treatment remains incomplete. Patient of gastritis not responding to the medicine may have gallstone, for which USG is mandatory to establish the cause.

A list of common pathological and laboratory test has been given below for the convenience and ready reference to our patients:

Sl. No.	Fundamental or Basic Test	Remark	Normal value
1)	Blood Sugar (Fasting)	Check once at least in a year. Check periodically, if diabetic.	80-100 mg/dl
	Blood Sugar (PP)	Necessary if Blood sugar level (Fasting) crosses the limit	100-140 mg/dl
2)	Blood Test for TC, DC, ESR, Hb%	Everybody should check once	Check w.r.t. normal limits
3)	Blood Pressure (Systolic and Diastolic)	Everybody should check once	Systolic < 120 mmHg Diastolic < 80 mmHg
4)	Glycosylated Haemoglobin (HbA1c)	Diabetic patients should check once in 6-8 months	Upto 7%
5)	Lipid Profile	Everybody should check once	Preferred LDL/ HDL Ratio = Upto 3.0
6)	Electrocardiogram (ECG)	Everybody should check once	Note the defect, if any
7)	T3, T4 and TSH	May be checked if indicated like weakness, lethargy, palpitation, hair loss, etc.	TSH = 0.3 to 3.0 mu/L

8)	Ultrasonography (USG) of whole abdomen	If indicated like pain in abdomen, menstrual problem, chronic gastritis or hyperacidity	Note the defect, if any. May indicate surgical treatment
9)	Blood Test for Uric Acid	For Arthritis Patients	Normal = 3.0-7.0 mg/dl
10)	Liver Function Test	Specially indicated in Jaundice	Jaundice if total bilirubin exceeds 1.5 mg/dl

It is always better that patients undergo the needful tests for Blood Sugar (Fasting) and Lipid Profile voluntarily from reputed laboratory and check their Blood Pressure before starting our medicines. This will not only enable early detection of Diabetes or Cardiovascular disease, which are common nowadays, but also will help to decide the dose of the medicine, taking in account of the defect, if any. Patients suffering from complex diseases with weakness and palpitation of heart should undergo test for Thyroid function in addition to above tests.

Blood Sugar and Lipid Profile Test may be termed as "Basic tests" which must be done by all of our patients especially who are above 30 years of age. If diabetes is detected, frequent test for Blood sugar is required along with intake of medicines, till the sugar-level comes down to normal.

BLOOD SUGAR AND LIPID PROFILE ARE THE BASIC TESTS WHICH OUR PATIENTS SHOULD DO BEFORE STARTING OUR TREATMENT

* * *

TIPS FOR TREATMENT OF PET ANIMALS AND BIRDS

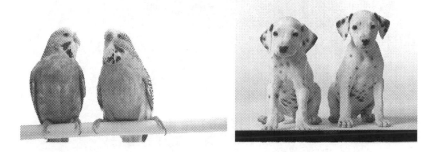

Animal lovers will be glad to know that our medicines are equally effective for keeping health of pet animals like cows, goats, dogs, etc. and pet birds like parrots, colourful birds, ducks, chicken, etc. All these creatures need not be fed with traditional medicines and artificial vitamins for treatment of their diseases, as well as for maintenance of their health.

During sickness of the pets, simply give few doses of "Booster" medicine by mixing it with their food or drinking water. Pets, animals or birds should be fed with few doses of "Bio-Tone Plus" in addition to above for weakness of nervous system.

These two multifarious medicines, if given occasionally and periodically (say once or twice in a week or month), will correct their metabolic disorder in a similar way as human being, and will help to maintain health of the pets.

SIMPLY APPLY FEW DOSES OF BIO-TONE PLUS AND BOOSTER FOR MAINTENANCE OF HEALTH OF YOUR PETS

---

*   *   *

GENETIC RELATIONSHIP BETWEEN DISEASE AND LONGEVITY

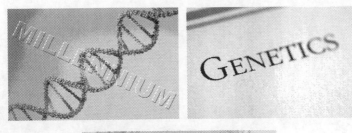

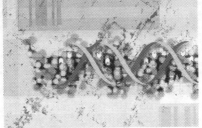

The human genome is stored on 23 pairs of chromosome and contains about 20,000 distinct genes. Human biology involves both genetic (inherited) and non-genetic (environmental) factors. In other words genetic disorders cause disease in combination with environmental factors such as lifestyle, diet and pollution. Genetic disorder may be associated with a single gene or multiple genes. In fact all diseases like diabetes, cardiovascular disease, cancer, asthma, migraine, schizophrenia, sickle cell anemia, retinitis pigmentosa, obesity, etc., have direct relationship with defective gene in the chromosome.

Another cause of the disease is associated with the length of the protective cap (telomeres) at the end of chromosome. Shorter telomeres cause poor health condition and aging. Special enzyme (telomerase) retards shortening of telomeres and prevents cell undergoing ageing effect. Shortening of telomere is an irreversible process. This explains why certain diseases are not curable unless gene therapy is adopted (unfortunately this therapy is still under primitive stage). While longevity or life-span depends on genome coding of an individual, the length of telomere denotes the condition of health with respect to chronological age.

Thus a man or woman of particular race or family having life-expectancy above 100 years will rarely suffer from any disease compared to an individual having 80 years of life-expectancy when both of them live under the same environmental condition. Thus the disease has direct relationship with the life-span (genetic clock) of the individual.

Conclusion:

In spite of the predominance of genome-coded life-span, our aim is to maintain the favorable condition of telomere-repairing enzyme i.e. telomerase. Bio-force stored in green chlorophyll and coloured pigments (bioflavonoid) can surprisingly keep telomerase enzyme more energetic to perform its duty, thus reducing risk or intensity of disease. Therefore, the keyword of health is "add more chlorophyll and coloured pigments" of nature in your daily life.

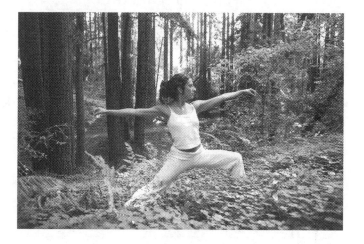

CHAPTER-4: DISEASE VS MEDICINE

EASYMEDICINE

QUICK REFERENCE OF MEDICINES FOR DISEASES

SEVERE TYPE OF VERTIGO
BIO-TONE PLUS (NORMALLY 2 DOSES/ DAY) + BOOSTER IN ABOUT 3:1 RATIO. ADDITIONALLY TAKE SHAKTI-RAJ & SUGAR-TABLET OR LIV-TREAT DAILY

OLD AGE PROBLEM, WEAKNESS OF NERVES
BIO-TONE PLUS & BOOSTER IN ABOUT 3:1 RATIO ADDITIONALLY TAKE SHAKTI-RAJ & SUGAR-TABLET OR LIV-TREAT REGULARLY

NERVE TONIC IN PARKINSON'S DISEASE
BIO-TONE PLUS & BOOSTER IN ABOUT 3:1 RATIO (TO BE TAKEN FOR LONG TERM) + SUGAR-TABLET OR LIV-TREAT & SHAKTI-RAJ (AFTER FOOD) + BIO-HERBS + DANTA-RAJ (BRUSH TWICE DAILY)

PREVENT LOSS OF MEMORY IN OLD AGE
BIO-TONE PLUS & BOOSTER IN ABOUT 3:1 RATIO ADDITIONALLY TAKE SUGAR-TABLET OR LIV-TREAT & SHAKTI-RAJ REGULARLY

MIGRAINE FOR MANY YEARS, HEADACHE
BIO-TONE PLUS & BOOSTER IN ABOUT 3:1 RATIO + FEVER COLD (REPEATEDLY DURING ATTACK) + SUGAR-TABLET OR LIV-TREAT & SHAKTI-RAJ (AFTER FOOD) + BIO-HERBS + DANTA-RAJ (BRUSH TWICE DAILY)

NERVE TONIC IN PSYCHIATRY DISORDER
BIO-TONE PLUS & BOOSTER IN ABOUT 3:1 RATIO (TO BE TAKEN FOR LONG TERM) + SUGAR-TABLET OR LIV-TREAT & SHAKTI-RAJ (AFTER FOOD) + BIO-HERBS + DANTA-RAJ (BRUSH TWICE DAILY)

MENTAL DEPRESSION, INSOMNIA
BIO-TONE PLUS & BOOSTER IN ABOUT 3:1 RATIO + SUGAR-TABLET OR LIV-TREAT & SHAKTI-RAJ (AFTER FOOD) + BIO-HERBS (TAKE PLENTY) + DANTA-RAJ (BRUSH BEFORE GOING TO SLEEP)

SEVERE, UNBEARABLE PAIN OF NERVES
APPLY BIO-TONE PLUS REPEATEDLY AT 15-20 MINUTES INTERVAL TILL CRISIS PERIOD IS OVER (PAIN MAY BE ANYWHERE IN THE BODY)

SEVERE COUGH, BRONCHITIS, VIRAL FEVER
BIO-TONE PLUS + BOOSTER 4-5 DOSES EACH TYPE REPEATEDLY ON THE VERY FIRST DAY AND THEREAFTER MAINTENANCE DOSE FOR FEW DAYS

SMOKERS' COUGH & CONGESTED LUNG
COUGH, PHLEGM & DUST ALLERGY EVEN ASTHMATIC TENDENCY: TAKE BIO-TONE PLUS & BOOSTER IN ABOUT 3:1 RATIO ON REGULAR BASIS

CHILDREN'S COMMON PROBLEMS, FEVER, COUGH, TONSILLITIS
BIO-TONE PLUS & BOOSTER. FEVER-COLD, STOMACH-STOOL, SHAKTI-RAJ AND SUGAR-TABLET OR LIV-TREAT AS APPLICABLE

CHILDREN'S HEALTH TONIC & MEMORY
BIO-TONE PLUS & BOOSTER (FOR GENERAL HEALTH, MEMORY & IMMUNITY) + SHAKTI-RAJ (FOR LIVER & EYE) + SUGAR-TABLET OR LIV-TREAT (FOR BILE) + BIO-HERBS (FOR DETOXIFICATION) + DANTA-RAJ (ORAL HYGIENE)

HIGH GRADE TONIC FOR PREGNANT MOTHERS
BIO-TONE PLUS & BOOSTER IN ABOUT 2:1 RATIO (FOR GENERAL HEALTH AS WELL AS FOR BABY'S IMMUNITY) + SHAKTI-RAJ & SUGAR-TABLET OR LIV-TREAT (AFTER FOOD) + BIO-HERBS + DANTA-RAJ

ACIDITY, GAS, FATTY LIVER DISEASE
BIO-TONE PLUS & BOOSTER + SHAKTI-RAJ & SUGAR-TABLET OR LIV-TREAT (AFTER FOOD) + BIO-HERBS (TAKE PLENTY) + DANTA-RAJ (ORAL HYGIENE)

DIARRHOEA, WATERY STOOL, VOMITING
SHAKTI-RAJ & MULTI-CARE MIXED TOGETHER IN WATER. ALTERNATIVELY TAKE STOMACH-STOOL IN REPEATED DOSES

BLEEDING PILES, FISTULA, CONSTIPATION
BIO-TONE PLUS & BOOSTER IN 2:1 OR 1:1 RATIO + SHAKTI-RAJ & SUGAR-TABLET OR LIV-TREAT (AFTER FOOD) + BIO-HERBS (TAKE PLENTY FOR NATURAL VITAMINS & FIBERS) + DANTA-RAJ (BRUSH TWICE DAILY)

LEVER TONIC, WEAKNESS IN DIGESTION
BIO-TONE PLUS & BOOSTER IN 2:1 OR 1:1 RATIO + SHAKTI-RAJ (FRUCTOSE ADDED) & SUGAR-TABLET OR LIV-TREAT (AFTER FOOD) + BIO-HERBS (FOR CONTIPATION) + DANTA-RAJ (BRUSH TWICE DAILY)

CARDIO-VASCULAR DISEASE, HIGH PRESSURE
BIO-TONE PLUS & BOOSTER IN 2:1 OR 1:1 RATIO + SHAKTI-RAJ & SUGAR-TABLET OR LIV-TREAT (AFTER FOOD) + BIO-HERBS (TO BE TAKEN PLENTY) + DANTA-RAJ + GREEN & COLOUR NATURAL PIGMENTS

DIABETES (TYPE 2), DIABETIC NEUROPATHY
REDUCED CALORIE INTAKE + SUGAR-TABLET + PLENTY OF BIO-HERBS + BIO-TONE PLUS & BOOSTER IN 2:1 OR 1:1 RATIO + DANTA-RAJ + JUICE OF PUMPKIN & *GULANCHA* + GREEN & COLOUR NATURAL PIGMENTS

PREVENT CANCER OR DIFFICULT DISEASES
BIO-TONE PLUS & BOOSTER IN 2:1 OR 1:1 RATIO + SHAKTI-RAJ & SUGAR-TABLET OR LIV-TREAT (AFTER FOOD) + BIO-HERBS (TAKE REGULARLY FOR FIBROUS DIET) + DANTA-RAJ (BRUSH TWICE DAILY)

ARTHRITIS, OSTEOARTHRITIS, GOUT
BIO-TONE PLUS & BOOSTER IN 2:1 OR 1:1 RATIO + SHAKTI-RAJ & SUGAR-TABLET OR LIV-TREAT (AFTER FOOD) + BIO-HERBS (TAKE PLENTY FOR DETOXIFICATION) + DANTA-RAJ (BRUSH TWICE DAILY) + MULTI-CARE (FOR PAIN)

CHRONIC HYPOTHYROIDISM, HYPERTHYROIDISM
BIO-TONE PLUS & BOOSTER IN 2:1 OR 1:1 RATIO + BIO-HERBS (PLENTY EVERYDAY) + SHAKTI-RAJ & SUGAR-TABLET OR LIV-TREAT (AFTER FOOD) + DANTA-RAJ (BRUSH TWICE DAILY)

MENSTRUAL PROBLEM, LEUCORRHOEA
BIO-TONE PLUS & BOOSTER IN 2:1 OR 1:1 RATIO. ADDITIONALLY TAKE BIO-HERBS (TAKE PLENTY) + SHAKTI-RAJ + SUGAR-TABLET OR LIV-TREAT

MINIMIZE OSTEOPOROSIS, MENOPAUSE PROBLEM
BIO-TONE PLUS + BOOSTER + BIO-HERBS (PLENTY) ADDITIONALLY TAKE SUGAR-TABLET OR LIV-TREAT + SHAKTI-RAJ + DANTA-RAJ

BLEEDING & SWELLING OF GUM, TOOTHACHE
APPLY MULTI-CARE REPEATEDLY AND BRUSH TWICE OR THRICE DAILY WITH DANTA-RAJ TOOTHPOWDER

PREVENT FALLING OF TEETH AT EARLY AGE
DANTA-RAJ (BRUSH TWICE DAILY) + MULTI-CARE (APPLY TWICE OR THRICE IN A WEEK) + INTERNAL MEDICINES BIO-TONE PLUS & BOOSTER + SUGAR-TABLET OR LIV-TREAT & SHAKTI-RAJ FOR GENERAL HEALTH

CUTS (BLEEDING), BURNS, INSECT BITE
APPLY SONALI ANTISEPTIC CREAM (EXTERNAL APPLICATION ONLY) + INTERNALLY TAKE FEVER-COLD 4-5 TIMES DAILY FOR 5-6 DAYS. ALTERNATIVELY APPLY MULTI-CARE ANTISEPTIC LOTION

PREVENTIVE MEDICINE FOR CATARACT OF EYE
BIO-TONE PLUS & BOOSTER IN ABOUT 3:1 RATIO (TAKE FOR LONG TERM) + SHAKTI-RAJ & SUGAR-TABLET OR LIV-TREAT (AFTER FOOD) + BIO-HERBS + DANTA-RAJ (BRUSH TWICE DAILY) + EYE-DROP OR MULTI-CARE

INCREASE LONGEVITY & AVIOD SURGERY
BIO-TONE PLUS & BOOSTER IN 3:1 RATIO (TAKE LIFELONG) + SHAKTI-RAJ & SUGAR-TABLET OR LIV-TREAT (AFTER FOOD) + BIO-HERBS (TAKE PLENTY) + DANTA-RAJ (BRUSH TWICE DAILY) + EYE-DROP OR MULTI-CARE

PREVENT DISEASE BY NATURAL MEDICINE
TAKE PLENTY OF GREEN CHLOROPHYLL AND COLOURED PIGMENTS AVAILABLE FROM GREEN LEAVES, COLOURED FRUITS AND NON-TOXIC COLOURED FLOWERS. THESE ARE THE WONDERFUL MEDICINES OF NATURE.

PREVENT DISEASE WITHOUT MEDICINE
UNDERGO FASTING FOR 1 OR 2 DAYS IN A MONTH TO KEEP AWAY MANY DISEASES IN LIFE. REMEMBER, OCCASIONAL FASTING ENHANCES IMMUNITY SYSTEM OF THE BODY.

*　　*　　*

CHAPTER-5: CHARTS AND TABLES

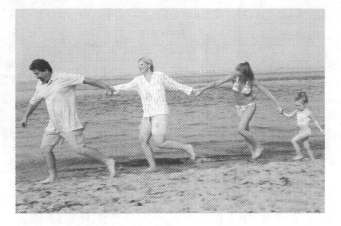

TABLE-I

GUIDELINE OF TREATMENT FOR COMPLICATED OR COMPLEX DISEASES

COMPARATIVE EFFECT OF MEDICINES UNDER "IDEAL AND EFFECTIVE MEDICATION"

GROUP	MEDICINE	RELATIVE VALUE OF MEDICATION
GROUP-I	REMEDY FOR NERVES, GLANDS AND VITAL ORGANS (KEEPS NERVES, GLANDS & ORGANS ACTIVE) **MEDICINE GROUP-I** **BIO-TONE PLUS (Triple)** **BOOSTER** (Take both medicines on regular basis)	EFFECT 60%

GROUP-II	REMEDY FOR DIGESTIVE SYSTEM (IMPROVES METABOLIC FUNCTION) **MEDICINE GROUP-II** **SUGAR-TABLET OR LIV-TREAT** **SHAKTI-RAJ (HONEY MIXED)** (Take both medicines after food)	EFFECT 10%
GROUP-III	REMEDY FOR DIRECT DETOXIFICATION (EXPELS TOXINS FROM BODY) **MEDICINE GROUP-III** **BIO-HERB NO. 1** **BIO-HERB NO. 2** (Take one type for few days, then alternate)	EFFECT 10%
GROUP-IV	REMEDY FOR MAGNESIUM DEFICIENCY (SUPPLEMENTS MAGNESIUM IN BODY) **MEDICINE GROUP-IV** **DANTA-RAJ** **(HERBAL TOOTHPOWDER)** (Brush twice daily)	EFFECT 5%

GROUP-V	INTAKE OF BIO-ENERGY (ENHANCES ACTIVITY OF MITOCHONDRIA OF CELL)	EFFECT
	B I O - E N E R G Y (BIOFLAVONOID) GROUP-V GREEN CHLOPHYLL OF NATURE (FROM FRESH CORIANDER LEAVES OR SIMILAR TYPE OF GREEN LEAVES) **COLOURED PIGMENTS (BIOFLAVONOID) OF NATURE** (FROM CARROT, BLACK GRAPES OR SIMILAR TYPES OF COLOURED FRUITS OR NON-TOXIC COLOURED FLOWERS) (Take plenty in empty stomach)	15%

**SUM TOTAL OF RELATIVE MEDICATION VALUE = 100%
MULTIPLY BY INDEX FACTOR (MAXIMUM VALUE = 1) TO
GET COMPLETE MEDICATION VALUE**

HOW TO CALCULATE NET OR EFFECTIVE MEDICATION VALUE?

Sl. No.	STEPS FOR CALCULATION
1)	MULTIPLY BY INDEX FACTOR (MAXIMUM VALUE=1) TO GET GROSS MEDICATION VALUE
•	GROSS MEDICATION VALUE (GMV): For example, if someone consumes only medicines of Group-I and II, his relative medication value (RMV) will be 70%. Now multiply by Index Factor which represents quantity or amount of medicine consumed. Suppose one consumes 60% of the recommended amount of medicine, his index factor (IF) will be 0.6. Hence Gross Medication Value (GMV) will be RM x IF = 0.7 x 0.6 = 0.42 = 42%.
2)	HOW TO CALCULATE THE NET MEDCATION VALUE? SIMPLY MULTIPLY BY AGE FACTOR.
•	NET MEDICATION VALUE (NMV): To calculate the Net Medication Value (NMV) we have to consider "Age Factor (AF)" which indicates "net utilization or efficiency of medicinal effect with respect to age". Thus a child will bear maximum value of 'age factor' whereas an old person will have least value of age factor. Let us take age factor as 1.0 for a child upto 10 years, reducing by 10% for increase of age by 10 years. An old person of 80 years age will thus have this factor 0.2, a person of 90 years will have only 0.1. For example a person of 80 years age will have NMV = 0.42 x 0.2 = 0.084 = 8.4% only compared to a child of 15 years age as 0.42 x 0.8 = 0.336 = 33.6%. Note that Net Medication Value greatly reduces with increase of age (for above calculation it is 4.0 times reduced for the old person when compared with the child. This explains why a child quickly responses to medicine than an old person with the same amount of medicine.

3)	ANOTHER EXAMPLE OF CALCULATION:
•	EXAMPLE CALCULATING NET MEDICATION VALUE (NMV):
	Another example—if someone consumes only medicines from Group-II and III, his relative medication value (RMV) will be 20%. Suppose one consumes 80% of the recommended amount of medicine, his Gross Medication Value (GMV) will be RM x IF = 0.2 x 0.8 = 0.16 = 16%.
	Considering a person of 70 years age consuming the medicine, his Net Medication Value will be 0.16 x 0.3 = 0.048 = 4.8% only, whereas a young man of 22 years age consuming the same amount of medicine will have NMV = 0.16 x 0.7 = 0.112 = 11.2%. This means the young man will be benefited by 2.3 times than the old person.
REMARK: GENETIC FACTORS HAVE NOT BEEN CONSIDERED HERE FOR SIMPLICITY OF CALCULATION.	

NET MEDICATION VALUE IS THE ACTUAL OR EFFECTIVE SCALE OF MEASUREMENT FOR MEDICATION. CALCULATE AND CHECK YOURSELF YOUR NET MEDICATION VALUE TO ANALYZE THE ACTUAL EFFECT OF MEDICATION.

ABOVE CALCULATION INDICATES THAT ONE SHOULD ACHEVE MAXIMUM "NET MEDICINAL VALUE" TO SUPPORT THE "IDEAL AND COMPLETE MEDICATION".

FOR COMPLEX DISEASES, ONE SHOULD THEREFORE CONSUME ALL MEDICINES REFERRED UNDER "GROUP-I TO V" MENTIONED ABOVE.

SAME MEDICINES ARE APPLICABLE FOR TREATMENT OF ALL TYPES OF CHRONIC DISEASES—NEUROLOGICAL DISEASES, ARTHRITIS, HIGH URIC ACID, GENERAL EYE PROBLEM, HEART DISEASE, CANCER, DIABETES, GASTRITIS, PILES, WEAK DIGESTION, FATTY LIVER DISEASE, SKIN DISEASE, THYROID, ASTHMA, BRONCHITIS, FEMALE DISEASE, PEDIATRIC DISEASE, OLD-AGE DISEASE AND SO ON.

For further details refer website: www.homemedicine.in

A COMMON SYSTEM OF TREATMENT FOR ALL COMPLEX DISEASES

CONCEPT OF "IDEAL AND COMPLETE MEDICATION" MUST BE APPLIED FOR TREATMENT OF DESTRUCTIVE DISEASE LIKE CANCER AND DIABETES

TABLE-II

GUIDELINE OF TREATMENT FOR INFANTS AND CHILDREN

DISEASE	MEDICINE	DIRECTION OF USE
Fever of all types	**First choice:** 1) Bio-Tone Plus (Triple) 2) Booster **Second choice:** 3) Fever-Cold 4) Stomach-Stool	a) Take Bio-Tone Plus & Booster repeatedly in alteration (say 2-3 doses each daily). b) Take Fever-Cold & Stomach-Stool repeatedly in alteration.
Diarrhea, Dysentery, Watery Stool, Vomiting, Indigestion	**First choice:** 1) Shakti-Raj & Multi-Care mixed together in water and take frequently. **Second choice:** 2) Stomach-Stool 3) Fever-Cold	a) Mix 8-10 caps Shakti-Raj & 5-6 droppers Multi-Care medicine in a glass of water and take frequently. b) Take Stomach-Stool repeatedly. c) In case of stomach problem with fever, take Fever-Cold & Stomach-Stool repeatedly in alteration.

Viral Fever, Flue, Malaria, Typhoid or Unknown type of Fever, Severe Tonsillitis, Throat Pain with High Fever, Cough, Asthma	<u>First choice:</u> 1) Bio-Tone Plus (Triple) 2) Booster <u>Second choice:</u> 3) Fever-Cold	a) Initially take large doses of Bio-Tone Plus & Booster repeatedly in alteration, say 3-4 doses each type. Later on take maintenance dose. Medicines are highly effective in all cases. b) Alternatively, repeated doses of Fever-Cold to be applied.
Food Allergy, Dust Allergy	<u>Best medicine:</u> 1) Bio-Tone Plus (Triple) 2) Booster <u>Supportive medicine</u>: 1) Shakti-Raj 2) Sugar-Tablet or Liv-Treat 3) Fever-Cold 4) Stomach-Stool	a) Bio-Tone Plus is compulsory medicine for all types of food and dust allergy and should be taken regularly for at least 1-2 years. b) Take Bio-Tone Plus and Booster in 3:1 or 2:1 ratio.

Growth, Nutrition, Immunity, Memory, Liver & General Problems	Compulsory medicine: 1) Bio-Tone Plus (Triple) 2) Booster Supportive medicine: 1) Shakti-Raj (tonic for nutrition) 2) Sugar-Tablet or Liv-Treat (correction of bile) 3) Bio-Herbs (natural vitamins and dietary fiber) 4) Danta-Raj (magnesium supplement) 5) Aqua-Fresh (for skin-care) 6) Herbal Eye-Drop (environmental pollution)	a) Bio-Tone Plus & Booster are high grade medicines for nerves, lymph and blood—improves memory and function of glands. b) Shakti-Raj improves liver function and provides nutrition; Sugar-Tablet or Liv-Treat corrects bile function, Bio-Herbs provide dietary fibers and Danta-Raj supplements magnesium. c) Aqua-Fresh protects skin from infection. Herbal Eye-Drop protects eye from air-pollution and microwave pollution.

BIO-TONE PLUS AND BOOSTER ARE EXCELLENT PREVENTIVE MEDICINES FOR MAJORITY OF PEDIATRIC DISEASES. MEDICINE UPGRADES IMMUNITY SYSTEM OF CHILDREN.

TABLE-III

IT IS EASY TO SELECT MEDICINES FOR CHRONIC AND COMPLICATED DISEASES

DISEASE MAY BE MANY, BUT MEDICINES ARE COMMON

GROUP	MEDICINE	DIRECTION OF USE
I	**BIO-TONE PLUS** (Triple) **BOOSTER**	Initially higher dose is required depending on severity of disease. Thereafter take 1-2 doses Bio-Tone Plus and 1 dose Booster daily.
II	**S H A K T I - R A J** (Honey Mixed) **SUGAR-TABLET OR LIV-TREAT**	Generally take 1-3 caps Shakti-Raj and 5-6 tablets Sugar-Tablet or Liv-Treat once or twice daily after food.
III	**BIO-HERB NO. 1 BIO-HERB NO. 2**	Take 1 type of Bio-Herb for few days and alternate with the other periodically. Take Bio-Herbs in sufficient quantity. Medicine may be taken at bedtime or in the morning. Take plenty of water.
IV	**DANTA-RAJ** (Toothpowder)	Brush teeth twice daily—at morning and night.
V	**GREEN CHLOROPHYLL COLOURED PIGMENTS (BIOFLAVONOID)**	Take plenty of fresh and unpreserved green leaves, coloured vegetables, fruits and non-toxic coloured flowers in un-cooked condition. Always take in empty stomach.

REMARKS:
a) Keep all the 7 nos. medicines of Group I to IV in your ready-stock.
b) It is better if both Bio-Tone Plus and Booster medicines are taken daily.
c) Green Chlorophyll and Coloured pigments (Bioflavonoid) must be used for treatment of all complicated diseases.

EASIEST WAY OF TREATMENT IS TO "JUST PICK UP" THE MEDICINES FROM OUR CLINIC AND BUILD-UP YOUR HOME-STOCK FOR DAILY USE → CONSULTATION IS NOT AT ALL NECESSARY BECAUSE MEDICINES ARE COMMON FOR ALL DISEASES → YOU NEED NOT WASTE YOUR VALUABLE TIME SEEKING OUR CONSULTATION.

TABLE-IV

HOW TO FIND OUT THE REASON OF FAILURE CHECK LIST FOR SELF-ASSESSMENT

IF YOUR RESULT IS UNSATISFACTORY, CHECK THE FOLLOWING: (PUT √ MARK ON YES/NO BELOW)

	REASON OF FAILURE	CHECKED
•	**Your case is basically surgical i.e. beyond scope of treatment under medicine.** Action: In case medicines do not respond, undergo pathological and surgical investigations.	YES/NO
•	**You have not taken adequate quantity of medicines. Your medication is incomplete.** Action: Take adequate doses of medicine daily, especially in acute condition. During crisis period, take large and repeated doses of Bio-Tone Plus and Booster medicine, high-grade tonics for nerve, gland and blood. Compute your "Net Medication Value" as per Table-I.	YES/NO
•	**You have not covered at least one medicine from each Group I to IV.** Action: Cover at least one medicine from each Group I to IV daily and alternate with balance medicines (preferably take both Bio-Tone Plus and Booster daily). Always keep all 8 nos. medicines in your ready home-stock.	YES/NO

•	**You have not used "Natural Medicines" in complicated diseases.** Action: Take Green Chlophyll and Coloured Pigments (Group V) available in Nature.	YES/NO
•	**Detoxification of your Body is probably incomplete.** Action: Take plenty of herbal medicines (Bio-Herbs) for complete detoxification of your body by direct method, through soft or loose stool. Take Bio-Tone Plus and Booster on regular basis to activate your internal organs to expel more toxins by indirect method.	YES/NO
•	**Your disease may be linked with "High Genetic factor" and "Emergency Condition".** Action: Avail modern system of medicine (allopathy) and facilities.	YES/NO
•	**Factors of "Diet" and "Exercise" might have played significant role. Restriction on diet in certain diseases (e.g. diabetes, kidney and heart disease) is essential. Similarly special exercise may be required for patients of Arthritis.** Action: Consult Specialist Doctor / Nutritionist / Physiotherapist.	YES/NO

INTERESTED PEOPLE SHOULD ALSO CALCULATE THE "GROSS MEDICATION VALUE" AND "NET MEDICATION VALUE" FROM TABLE-I.

THIS WILL ENABLE THEM TO DO THE SELF-ASSESSMENT MORE ACCURATELY AND LOGICALLY

TABLE-V

KEEP YOURSELF HEALTHY, INCREASE LONGEVITY, AVOID SURGERY IN LIFE AND PREVENT DREADFUL AND COMPLICATED DISEASES

Use "GENERAL MEDICINES" under GROUP I to IV:
Medicines for Nerves, Glands and Vital Organs: BIO-TONE PLUS and BOOSTER
Medicines to improve Digestive Function: SUGAR-TABLET OR LIV-TREAT and SHAKTI-RAJ
Medicines for direct Detoxification of Body: BIO-HERB NOS. 1 & 2
Medicines to maintain Hygiene of Mouth: DANTA-RAJ and MULTI-CARE
Use NATURAL MEDICINE (Green Chlorophyll and Coloured Pigments), AQUA-FRESH and HERBAL EYE-DROP to complete the cycle for "MAINTENANCE OF HEALTH".

Our aim is to minimize your visit at our Clinic to seek Doctor's Consultation. Take moderate amount of above "Medicines" everyday as "Health Tonic" to get rid of Complicated Disease and avoid Surgery in your life. Pay a little attention on your Health to keep away many troubles in life. Remember, Health is Wealth— "Prevention is always better than Cure".

Cure yourself or remain healthy by simple treatment with a combination of Herbal, Homeopathy, Biochemic and Ayurvedic Medicines. Note that all medicines are Non-toxic, Multifarious type and applicable for people of all ages—children, adult and old.

REFER LIST "DISEASE VS MEDICINE" FOR EASY AND SIMPLE SOLUTION OF YOUR PROBLEMS

READ "EASYMEDICINE" BOOK THOROUGHLY. PATIENTS NEED NOT COME TO OUR CLINIC FOR CONSULTATION. JUST PICK-UP THE MEDICINES FROM THE CLINIC AND START YOUR OWN TREATMENT.

TABLE-VI

STANDARD PRESCRIPTION FOR ANY COMPLEX DISEASE

Name of Patient   Age   Date

Address & Telephone No.

Complaint of / Problem:

LIST OF MEDICINE: PUT √ MARK AS APPLICABLE

☐ BIO-TONE PLUS (Triple / Double)-Packet

☐ BOOSTER-Packet

☐ SUGAR-TABLET (Herbal)

☐ LIV-TREAT Herbal Tablet

☐ SHAKTI-RAJ Digestive Tonic

☐ BIO-HERB NO. 1 (Biochemic & Herbs)

☐ BIO-HERB NO. 2 (Biochemic & Herbs)

☐ DANTA-RAJ Herbal Toothpowder

☐ MULTI-CARE Antiseptic Lotion

☐ AQUA-FRESH Herbal Bath

☐ HERBAL EYE-DROP

☐ FEVER-COLD Liquid

☐ STOMACH-STOOL Liquid

☐ SONALI Herbal Antiseptic Cream

- Read EASYMEDICINE Book for detail and application of medicines.

- Refill your Home-stock medicines as and when required.

- Remember, disease may be many but medicines are same.

- Five "Basic Cares" can prevent complex and dreadful diseases; avoid hospitalization and surgery in life—"Mouth-care", "Stomach-care", "Detoxification", "Skin-care" & "Eye-care".

ADVICE ON MEDICINE & DIET:

ADVICE FOR BASIC MEDICAL TEST:

1) Lipid Profile	2) Blood Pressure
3) Blood Sugar	4) HbA1c
5) Liver Function	6) T3, T4, TSH
7) Blood (Routine)	8) USG (whole abdomen)

_____

Signature

TABLE-VII

SCHEMA FOR STANDARD PREVENTIVE HOME-MEDICINES

Five "Basic Cares" can prevent complex & dreadful diseases; avoids hospitalization and surgery in life → "Mouth-care", "Stomach-care", "Detoxification", "Skin-care" & "Eye-care".

Sl. No.	Name of the Medicine	How it Prevents Disease	Diseases Prevented
1)	"BIO-TONE PLUS" (Triple / Double) & "BOOSTER"	Medicine for Nervous System and Glands → Increases immunity system of the body. Moderate dose (say 1 week for child & 2 weeks for adult, in a month) is sufficient to increase immunity potential.	Disease of nerves, gland, eye, arthritis, cold & cough, children & female disease, high pressure, thyroid, old age problems, etc. Applicable for all ages → children to very old persons. Youngsters can easily get rid of spectacles.
2)	"SUGAR-TABLET" OR "LIV-TREAT" OR "SHAKTI-RAJ"	High-grade medicine for Liver. Keeps the food relatively alkaline (i.e. less acidic w.r.t. gastric juice having pH = 1 to 3) and prevents metabolic disorder. Helps digestion.	Acidity, weakness of digestion, fatty liver disease, skin disease, etc. Shakti-Raj promotes growth & nutrition of children. Sugar-Tablet prevents diabetes, skin disease, acidity & gas.

3)	"BIO-HERB NO. 1" OR "BIO-HERB NO. 2"	Provides Dietary Fiber and Biochemic medicine. Detoxifies by expelling toxins from body. Helps absorption of nutrients by small intestine.	Prevents constipation, high cholesterol, high pressure, thyroid, arthritis, skin disease, etc. High-grade preventive medicine for cancer & complex diseases.
4)	"DANTA-RAJ" Toothpowder	Avoids Fluoride Poisoning. Fluorine (F) has the highest electron affinity and forms stable compounds. Reacts with Ca, Mg, Fe and other +ve ions of the body, causing dysfunction of useful enzymes.	Prevents arthritis, cataract of eye (of diabetic patients), acidity & weakness of digestion, high-grade tonic for optic nerve. Maintains normal activity of enzymes and indirectly improves immunity system.

Using above Four types medicines on regular basis, one can easily save lot of money and time by avoiding hospitalization and surgery in life such as gall-stone, bypass surgery, fitment of pacemaker, etc. Learn the "easiest method" to prevent Cancer & Cardiovascular disease.

5)	MULTI-CARE	Apply twice or thrice in a week to keep gum healthy and strong.	Prevents all types of dental & mouth problems. Prevents skin infection.
6)	AQUA-FRESH	Protects skin especially for babies & children. High-grade cosmetic for ladies.	Prevents skin disease, itching, eczema and fungal infection. Note: Alternatively use Multi-Care.
7)	HERBAL EYE-DROP	Protects eye from microwave radiation and relieves strain.	Keeps eye free from disease & cataract. Note: Alternatively use Multi-Care or Aqua-Fresh (refer Table-X).

Note the Schema for "state-of-the-art" on Preventive Medicine. Remember "Prevention is always better than cure". Our aim is to minimize the expenditure on treatment of serious or dreadful diseases by adopting "Preventive Medicine" on grass-root level.

S. B. HEALTH GUIDE IS THE PIONEER IN PREVENTIVE MEDICINES.

THE MOST IMPORTANT ASPECT FOR MAINTENANCE OF HEALTH IS EXTENSIVE USE OF *NATURAL MEDICINES* I.E. GREEN CHLOROPHYLL AND COLOURED PIGMENTS OF NATURE. YOU CAN PREVENT AT LEAST 50% DISEASE IN LIFE BY TAKING *NATURAL MEDICINES*. MEDICINES REFERRED ABOVE ARE ACTUALLY MEANT FOR THE PEOPLE WHO ARE NOT FAMILIAR WITH THE *AMAZING POWER OF NATURAL MEDICINES*. KEEP YOURSELF PRACTICALLY DISEASE-FREE BY TAKING *NATURAL MEDICINES!*

NON-TOXIC COLOURED FLOWERS ARE HIGHLY RECOMMENDED FOR USE AS PREVENTIVE *NATURAL MEDICINE*. ADD FEW PIECES OF THE SAME IN YOUR REGULAR DIET. INCIDENTALLY IT IS ALSO THE BEST AND CHEAPEST FORM OF *NATURAL MEDICINE!*

FEW PIECES OF GREEN *NEEM* LEAVES AND RAW-GARLIC MAY ALSO BE TAKEN ON REGULAR BASIS TO KEEP AWAY MANY DISEASES IN LIFE.

TABLE-VIII

ADVANTAGES OF EASYMEDICINE IN
FAMILY-TREATMENT

	ADVANTAGES		USER-FRIENDLY APPLICATION IN FAMILY-TREATMENT
•	EASY to remember, easy to learn and easy to apply.	:	Read thoroughly "EASYMEDICINE" Book and refer website www.homemedicine.in. For comparative value of different medicines, refer Table-I. For quick reference, see "Disease Vs Medicine".
•	EASY to consume and easy to medicate.	:	Busy people should carry 1-2 packets of Bio-Tone Plus and Booster (weighing only few milligrams) in their briefcase and consume medicine anytime. These two medicines will cover about 60% of total medication value.
•	EASY to carry in traveler's kit for acute problems like viral fever, severe throat infection, bronchitis, etc.	:	Always keep few packets of Bio-Tone Plus and Booster in your briefcase before you commence travel—your journey will be trouble-free. These medicines are to be taken daily by you and your family to increase immunity and avoid unwanted problems during journey.
•	EASY to cover crisis management, especially in your tour.	:	Apply Bio-Tone Plus and Booster repeatedly at 15-20 minutes interval, till your crisis period is over. Thereafter take your own decision.
•	EASY to cover all diseases (except surgery) with few medicines.	:	Bio-Tone Plus and Booster are multifarious medicine and cover almost all diseases. Consume these two medicines blindly on regular basis.

• EASY to deal with all types of non-surgical diseases of children.	:	Apply Bio-Tone Plus and Booster in 1:1 ratio daily in any type of disease of the children. Apply blindly. For acute problems like high-fever, tonsillitis, etc., apply multiple doses daily.
• EASY to deal with all types of Female diseases and Gynecological problems.	:	Apply Bio-Tone Plus and Booster in 2:1 or 1:1 ratio daily in any type of Female disease. Take 1-2 doses each type daily. Additionally take BH, STLT, SR and DR.
• EASY to deal with or prevent complex diseases of old people.	:	Take 1-2 doses Bio-Tone Plus and Booster daily in 3:1 ratio from 50 years age and continue for whole life. Additionally use BH, STLT, SR, DR and ED.
• EASY to treat all neurological problems like vertigo, migraine, epilepsy, Parkinson's disease, sciatica, severe nerve-pain, etc.	:	Blindly take nerve tonic Bio-Tone Plus and Booster daily, preferably in 3:1 ratio and continue the medicine. Additionally take BH, STLT, SR and DR.\n\nFor severe and unbearable type of nerve pain, apply Bio-Tone Plus repeatedly at 15-30 minutes interval till crisis period is over.
• EASY to treat lymph-blood related diseases like cardiovascular disease, thyroid, swelling of glands, breast and uterine tumour, immunity deficiency, etc.	:	Take Bio-Tone Plus and Booster daily on regular basis in 2:1 or 1:1 ratio and continue the medicine. Additionally take STLT, SR and DR. Plenty of BH must be taken for detoxification. Take chlorophyll and coloured fruits in empty stomach.
• EASY to cure all types of skin disease.	:	Take Bio-Tone Plus and Booster daily in 1:1 ratio and continue the medicine. Additionally take STLT, SR, BH (take plenty) and DR. Take chlorophyll in empty stomach. Apply Multi-Care or Aqua-Fresh on skin for itching or irritation.

• EASY to treat constipation and all stomach problems like acidity, gas, piles, etc.	:	Bio-Tone Plus and Booster are high-grade medicine to remove constipation. Take on regular basis. Take plenty of BH and drink sufficient water. Additionally take STLT, SR and DR.
• EASY to treat destructive disease like cancer and diabetes.	:	Take high doses Bio-Tone Plus and Booster, say 2-4 doses of each medicine daily. Take 8-10 Sugar-Tablet daily. It is compulsory to take 2-3 glasses juice of coriander leaves, pumpkin and *gulancha* in empty stomach in the morning and evening. Coloured fruits must be added in juice for cancer patients. Never take the juice after meals.
• EASY to avoid surgery in life, lead disease-free life, increase longevity.	:	Bio-Tone Plus and Booster are high-grade medicine to build-up immunity. Take on regular basis. Take plenty of BH. Additionally take STLT, SR, DR and ED.
• EASY and user-friendly type medicine, common medicine for multiple diseases	:	There are limited numbers of medicines in our system. Medicines are of "multifarious" in action and cover wide range of diseases. Just build-up your home-stock and blindly apply the medicines in any disease, as per the guideline of this book. Thus the same medicine will practically cover array of complex diseases—you need not think of individual disease!
• EASY availability of medicine by Courier.	:	Home delivery is available in local area. For other places in India or abroad, medicines are sent to the patients through Courier Service. Full address, pin code and telephone or mobile number is to be given for this purpose, with name of the patient and disease. E-mail the requisite information to initiate delivery action.

<u>Abbreviations used:</u>

STLT: Sugar-Tablet or Liv-Treat, SR: Shakti-Raj, BH: Bio-Herb No. 1 or 2, DR: Danta-Raj, ED: Eye-Drop.

TABLE-IX

TECHNICAL BENEFIT OF EASYMEDICINE IN FAMILY-TREATMENT

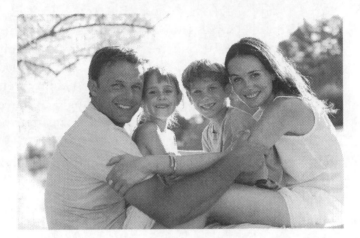

1)	There are only few basic medicines (mainly 7 medicines) by which one can treat and cover wide range of complex diseases. i) **Remedies for Nerve, Glands & Vital Organs**—"Bio-Tone Plus (Triple or Double Strength)" & "Booster", ii) **Fibrous remedies** for detoxification—"Bio-Herb No. 1 or 2", iii) **Liver & Stomach remedies**—"Shakti-Raj" or "Sugar-Tablet" or "Liv-Treat", iv) For **hygiene of Mouth**—"Danta-Raj" & "Multi-Care" and v) For **hygiene of Eye**—"Herbal Eye-Drop". Limited medicines means less confusion and user-friendly in respect of application of medicines. Therefore, **family-treatment** can be blindly carried out by using limited number of medicines for widest range of diseases without getting confused and seeking doctor's help. It is also the **easiest method of home-treatment** for multiple or complex disease. Additionally it can be used as **Preventive Medicine** for dreadful diseases, if continued for long.

2)	Medicines work on principle of **"Set Theory"**. The basic domains are **"Liver and Nerves"**. Liver is responsible for all metabolic disorder such as high cholesterol, high uric acid, digestive disorder and what not. It regulates purity of blood which is the main constituent of body. On the other hand Nerves control the whole body function. It is analogous to an electric cable: when electricity is passed—it becomes live, otherwise it is dead. Similarly the body without nervous system is meaningless. Therefore, one has to treat both LIVER and NERVES. The **medicines cover both.** Therefore, one need not **scratch his head to treat the patient** especially for complex disease. This is the advantage of set theory (analogous to modern concept of mathematics). The concept of Liver and Nerve is applied under the system of **family-treatment**.
3)	Nature follows **"Straight Line"** OR **"Path of Least Resistance"**. The concept of **home-treatment** is based on application of medicine instantly at the time of onset of disease without going for Physiological and Pathological examination. In case of failure of medicine, physiological and pathological check up should be started. Therefore, **try first with "Medicine"** without wasting **time and money** for initial laboratory test. Application of medicine at **"Zero Hour"** will simplify the case, especially where virus or bacteria multiply in GP series (however, laboratory tests are **essential** in **surgery-oriented diseases** such as gallstone or kidney stone or permanent deformation of tissue).
4)	The whole process of treatment is based on **"Vector Process"**. When one becomes sick, the motto is to treat him in most simple way (unless it is an emergency type). It is a Vector process having specific "Direction" or target i.e. "Cure" by **application of medicine.** Instead of going through straight process, we apply **zigzag process** by undergoing **pathological and laboratory tests** (which are termed as "Non-vector"). Above difference is analogous to Speed and Velocity in Physics—one is directionless whereas other is having specific direction. We therefore, suggest **applying medicines first** under **family-treatment**. Unfortunately we often follow the "zigzag" path of treatment which is purely Non-vector.

5)	Guideline for User-friendly System of Medicine and Treatment is elaborated in detail in the book "EASYMEDICINE". The book is written in most simple way, based on the knowledge of advanced science, viz. Cause of Disease, Biochemistry, Nutrition, Genetic Relationship with Disease and Analytical Logic. Refer the book and learn the **simplified but most effective system of home-treatment or family-treatment**. By keeping some home-stock of medicines, one can treat chronic and complex disease as well as some acute disease without wasting time for selection of medicine or pathological investigation. Thus one can **get rid of majority of problems with little or no effort**. It is however to be remembered that our treatment does not cover surgery, emergency or high-order genetic diseases for which we always recommend treatment through allopathic doctors or specialists.

TABLE-X

PRIMARY AND SECONDARY MEDICINES FOR HOME-TREATMENT

It is to be noted that certain medicines are called "Basic or Primary medicines" whereas rest are the "Derivatives or Secondary medicines". Thus by knowing application of medicines, one can easily reduce the variety of home-stock. For example Aqua-Fresh and Eye-Drop can be replaced by keeping Multi-Care lotion. Similarly Liv-Treat can be replaced by keeping Sugar-Tablet. Fever-Cold can also be replaced by deep-acting medicines Bio-Tone Plus and Booster. Following chart differentiates between primary and secondary medicines and indicates how one medicine can be replaced by another.

Sl. No.	Name of the Medicine	Type of Medicine	Remark on Replacement of Medicine
1)	BIO-TONE PLUS (Triple or Double Strength)	Basic or Primary Medicine	Basic medicine for nerve, glands and internal organs. For acute and chronic disease. Bio-Tone Plus acts more on nerves and Booster acts more on glands. Dose is to be decided depending on the disease-force. It is better to take the medicines in combination.
2)	BOOSTER	—DO—	
3)	SHAKTI-RAJ	—DO—	Covers more on digestive system and eye. However sugar tablet alone can cover the digestive problems and in this case Shakti-Raj can be replaced by Sugar-Tablet.

4)	SUGAR-TABLET	Basic or Primary Medicine	Essential for digestive problems. Sugar-Tablet should be used for all complicated cases. For practical purpose Liv-Treat can be replaced by Sugar-Tablet.
5)	LIV-TREAT	Derivative or Secondary Medicine	
6)	BIO-HERB NO. 1	Basic or Primary Medicine	Provides dietary fiber—essential for all chronic diseases. Either one of the medicines can be taken—however it is better to alternate the two.
7)	BIO-HERB NO. 2	—DO—	
8)	MULTI-CARE	Basic or Primary Medicine	Multi-Care and Aqua-Fresh are antiseptic and painkilling. Aqua-Fresh is a diluted variety of Multi-Care and can be eliminated from Home-stock list.
9)	AQUA-FRESH	Derivative or Secondary Medicine	
10)	H E R B A L EYE-DROP	—DO—	Herbal Eye-Drop is a further diluted variety of Aqua-Fresh. Few drops of Multi-Care or 2-3 droppers Aqua-Fresh mixed in a cup of water have the same effect on eye. Direct application of 1-2 drops Multi-Care or Aqua-Fresh on eyes is also recommended. Thus conventional Eye-Drop can be totally eliminated. However for eye disease additionally take Bio-Tone Plus and Booster.
11)	DANTA-RAJ	Basic or Primary Medicine	Covers hygiene of mouth and reduces stomach problems.

12)	FEVER-COLD	Derivative or Secondary Medicine	Bio-Tone Plus and Booster must be used in complicated cases. Thus Fever-Cold can be eliminated.
13)	STOMACH-STOOL	Sometimes Primary and sometimes Secondary	For loose motion or vomiting acts as primary, but for chronic stomach problems Sugar-Tablet acts better. Thus Stomach-Stool can be partially replaced by other medicine.
14)	SONALI	—DO—	Multi-Care covers almost all actions of Sonali. However in case of bites from poisonous insects, Sonali is practically the only remedy.

SELECT YOUR MEDICINE OR HOME-STOCK BY REDUCING VARIETY OF MEDICNES. PRACTICALLY 7-8 MEDICINES WILL BE SUFFICIENT FOR HOME-TREATMENT. SURGERY, EMERGENCY AND HIGH-ORDER GENETIC DISEASES ARE HOWEVER, TO BE DEALT BY ALLOPATHIC SPECIALIST DOCTORS.

CHAPTER-6: SUMMARY OF EASYMEDICINE

EASY TREATMENT
HOME-TREATMENT FOR COMPLEX
DISEASE

After the age of 30-40 years, we slowly become victim of complex or multiple diseases. At our earlier age we might have suffered from one or two diseases, but time comes when we become victim of a group of chronic diseases such as acidity, gas, constipation, weakness of digestion, fatty liver disease, piles, arthritis, high uric acid, high blood pressure, high cholesterol, hypo or hyper thyroidism, chronic cold and cough, skin disease, nerve-disease and so on. During menopause, women suffer from nerve-pain, sciatica, osteoarthritis, osteoporosis and many other diseases.

How to treat yourself especially when you are suffering from multiple or array of diseases? Will you take medicine for each and every disease and make a big list of medicine? Don't worry—you can treat complex disease in most simple way.

Treatment—First step of treatment begins with mouth and stomach. Brush teeth twice daily with DANTA-RAJ toothpowder. Apply 2-3 drops MULTI-CARE lotion on gum—gently rub by finger and swallow the medicine after application on gum. Take plenty of BIO-HERB 1 or 2 at bedtime and drink sufficient water in empty stomach in the morning. Toxins like arsenic, fluoride, pesticide, etc. will come out of body through soft or liquid stool—thus purifying your blood through detoxification. Take SHAKTI-RAJ and SUGAR-TABLET or LIV-TREAT for better digestion and improvement of liver-function. To improve the function of nerves and glands take BIO-TONE PLUS and

BOOSTER say 10-15 days in month. For eye problem or hygiene of skin, use HERBAL EYE-DROP and AQUA-FRESH respectively. Take limited food, more green leaves (Chlorophyll), vegetables, fresh fruits and non-toxic coloured flowers than fish or meat. Treat for blood sugar separately with special care.

By this way you can slowly get rid of disease within 3-4 months and able to keep yourself away from cluster of medicines. Remember this standard method of home-treatment for non-surgery type chronic and complex disease.

PREVENTIVE MEDICINE
FOR INCURABLE DISEASE

We are not familiar with the term "Preventive Medicine" in present system of treatment. In fact its application is limited to vaccination for small pox, polio and few other diseases. But there is no vaccine for dreadful diseases like cancer, AIDS, diabetes, arthritis and cardiovascular disease. These diseases are spreading like epidemic and we are spending huge amount of money for treatment of the same. No curative treatment is so far developed for these diseases. As a result doctors are often humiliated. But it is easy to prevent dreadful diseases by simple method of medication. Eliminate the cause of disease by expelling accumulated toxins from your body—you need to detoxify yourself everyday or on regular basis.

Take plenty of BIO-HERB 1 or 2 at bedtime and drink sufficient water early in the morning in empty stomach. The toxins accumulated in your body will come out through soft or liquid stool. Thus blood will be purified and you will get rid of toxin accumulated in your body. Brush your teeth twice daily by DANTA-RAJ toothpowder. Apply 2-3 drops MULTI-CARE lotion on gum—gently rub by finger and swallow the medicine after application on gum. Take SHAKTI-RAJ and SUGAR-TABLET or LIV-TREAT for better digestion and effective functioning of liver. For tonic of nerve and gland, take BIO-TONE PLUS and BOOSTER say 10-12 days in a month. To prevent eye disease or skin disease, add HERBAL

189

EYE-DROP and AQUA-FRESH respectively. Take limited food, more green leaves (Chlorophyll), vegetables, fresh fruits and non-toxic coloured flowers than fish or meat.

By this way one can easily prevent dreadful diseases with the help of few medicines only. It is better and economic to prevent disease by adopting "Preventive Medicine" than to actually suffer from disease. A little awareness on health and preventive system of treatment will practically keep your family free from disease.

Remember the old proverb—"Prevention is better than cure".

MOUTH & STOMACH CARE
THE FIRST STEP FOR ANY TREATMENT

Keyword of treatment for complex disease is cleanliness of mouth & teeth and expelling accumulated toxins from the body. Mouth and teeth must be kept bacteria-free and bowels should be cleared on regular basis to function the digestive system in a better way.

Brush your teeth by using DANTA-RAJ toothpowder twice daily and apply 2-3 drops MULTI-CARE antiseptic herbal lotion on your gum—gently rub by your finger and swallow the medicine. You will be surprised to note that one-third of stomach problem has been diminished—after all mouth is the starting point of the digestive system.

Take plenty of Biochemic-mixed herbal medicine BIO-HERB No. 1 or 2 at bedtime and drink sufficient water early in the morning in empty stomach. Toxins (arsenic, fluoride, pesticide, etc.) of your body will be expelled through soft or liquid stool by detoxification. Take SUGAR-TABLET or LIV-TREAT for better digestion and improvement of liver-function.

By this way you will find great improvement on any type of complex disease—high pressure, high cholesterol, high uric acid, arthritis, fatty liver disease, thyroid, constipation, bleeding of piles, skin disease and so on. In this process, blood will be purified and you will feel overall comfort.

BIO-TONE PLUS & BOOSTER
MEDICINE FOR APPLICATION IN ALL DISEASE

- Deep-acting special ayurvedic medicine for diseases related to Nerves and Glands • Acute and Chronic Vertigo, Nerve-pain, Sciatica, Headache, Migraine, Weakness of nerves, Eye-disease, Parkinson's disease, Insomnia and many other nerve-related disease • Swelling of Tonsils & Glands, Chronic Cold & Cough, Fever of small children as well as adults • Menstrual pain of young girls, Female disease.

- High-grade medicine for all Respiratory problems • Severe cold & cough, Tonsillitis, Bronchitis, Pneumonia, Throat infection, Viral fever, etc. • Cures faster than any other medicine, take repeatedly • Excellent medicine for High-pressure, High-cholesterol, Thyroid, Arthritis, Bleeding Piles, Fistula, Frozen shoulder, etc. (additionally take plenty of BIO-HERB 1 or 2).

- Medicines are having wide range of action—act on nerves, muscle, bone, blood and all internal organs such as liver, heart, kidney, eye and so on • Corrects disharmony of nervous system, lymphatic system and blood or circulatory system • Improves memory, immunity and eye-sight of children (additionally take SHAKTI-RAJ) • Best medicine for aged people for maintenance of health.

- High-grade preventive as well as curative medicine for all ages—from children to very old people • Essential medicine for application in all disease—should be kept as family-stock for home-treatment.

- For maintenance of health take BIO-TONE PLUS and BOOSTER (say 10-12 doses in a month) along with the General medicines i.e. BIO-HERB 1 or 2, SHAKTI-RAJ, SUGAR-TABLET or LIV-TREAT.

BIO-HERB NO. 1 & BIO-HERB NO. 2 MEDICINE FOR DETOXIFICATION

- Biochemic-mixed Herbal medicine for treatment of all diseases and maintenance of health • High-grade medicine for Constipation, Piles, High Pressure, High Cholesterol, Heart-disease, Arthritis, Frozen Shoulder, Uric Acid, Osteoarthritis, Thyroid, Skin disease, Obesity and many other problems.

- BIO-HERBs are the high-grade medicine for detoxification • Expels toxins from the body accumulated through pesticides, air, water and chemical pollution • Effective medicine for Arsenic and Fluoride Poisoning • Preventive Medicine for dreadful diseases if taken on regular basis • Regular intake of medicine will surely increase longevity—it is better to continue the medicine for lifelong.

- For treatment of any complex and multiple disease, take plenty of BIO-HERB 1 or 2 at bedtime and drink sufficient water in empty stomach in the morning • Toxins like arsenic, fluoride, pesticide, etc. will come out of your body through soft or liquid stool • Additionally use DANTA-RAJ twice daily, MULTI-CARE, SHAKTI-RAJ, SUGAR-TABLET or LIV-TREAT • Also take 10-15 doses BIO-TONE PLUS and BOOSTER in a month • Thus your treatment is simplified and you will feel much better within 3-4 months.

DANTA-RAJ HERBAL MEDICINE FOR MOUTH & TEETH

- Prevents diseases of Gum & Teeth • Pyorrhea • Foul Breath • Bleeding of Gum • Toothache • Ulcer on mouth • Increases longevity of Teeth (should not fall before 70-75 years age, unless there is blood sugar) • Regular use maintains Salivary Glands active and helps preventing many diseases • No perfume or frothing chemical used in it and salivary glands are thus protected • Young generation must use DANTA-RAJ herbal toothpowder and MULTI-CARE lotion for protection of salivary glands, thus avoiding disease like arthritis, diabetes, high blood pressure, high uric acid, etc. at their middle age.

- Danta-Raj also marginally reduces digestion problem such as acidity and gastritis • Swallow little bit of powder in case slight acidity is felt in stomach • An effective medicine for keeping optic nerves healthy, thus preventing many types of eye diseases (additionally take BIO-TONE PLUS, BOOSTER and SHAKTI-RAJ).

- Use hard quality of brush for brushing—preferably twice daily • Dental surgery may be needed if cavity exists on tooth • Store the medicine in cool place—do not expose to heat or sun.

SHAKTI-RAJ TONIC
MEDICINE FOR LIVER, EYE & DIGESTION

- An useful tonic for digestive system and general maintenance of health • Acidity, indigestion, gas, joint-pain, high uric-acid, osteoarthritis, high cholesterol, bleeding piles, varicose vein, skin disease, fatty lever disease, heart disease • Take 1-2 caps medicine daily to reduce risk of malaria and mosquito-borne diseases • Blood-purifier, improves circulation and prevents formation of clots in the blood • In summer, it cools down the body and brings comfort • Prevents tumour and warts • Action of the medicine is anti-cancerous if taken regularly • Medicine is of sour taste; hence some water may be added while taking the same.

- A high-grade medicine for all types of eye disease, especially glaucoma (take BIO-TONE PLUS & BOOSTER for 10-15 days in a month) • In chronic disease, additionally use DANTA-RAJ twice daily, apply MULTI-CARE on gum, take plenty of BIO-HERB to expel accumulated toxin from your body and SUGAR-TABLET or LIV-TREAT to improve digestion • In case of over-eating, it reduces uneasiness of the stomach.

• An essential health tonic for school-children • Improves memory, eye-sight and upgrades nutrition (additionally take few doses of BIO-TONE PLUS & BOOSTER on regular basis).

SUGAR-TABLET & LIV-TREAT
MEDICINE FOR LIVER & BILE FUNCTION

• Powerful herbal medicines for treatment of all diseases related to weakness of liver such as acidity, gas, indigestion, especially after suffering from Jaundice • Bleeding of Piles, High-pressure, High-cholesterol, Skin disease, Fatty liver disease, etc. (additionally take BIO-TONE PLUS & BOOSTER) • An excellent remedy for Chronic dysentery, for many years • Reduces acidic property of food which is the underlying cause of many disease • Essential medicine for regulation of bile and treatment for liver-related diseases.

• Take 5-6 tablets after meal or dinner—medicine is of bitter taste, swallow with water • To expel toxin from your body additionally take plenty of BIO-HERB 1 or 2 at bedtime and drink sufficient water in empty stomach early in the morning.

• Note that SUGAR-TABLET is more powerful than LIV-TREAT; it marginally reduces blood sugar and minimizes almost all stomach problems • SUGAR-TABLET is essential for treatment of skin disease (additionally take BIO-TONE PLUS, BOOSTER and Chlorophyll) • Medicine should be taken by diabetic as well as non-diabetic people—an essential medicine for the family.

MULTI-CARE LOTION
ANTISEPTIC MEDICINE FOR MULTIPURPOSE USE

- Powerful antiseptic herbal lotion for bleeding from cuts and wounds—apply on the affected area to stop infection and pus formation • Apply on burns—no blister will appear • Excellent medicine for Pyorrhea, Swelling of gum, Toothache, Bleeding from gum, Spongy gum, Foul smell from mouth, Ulcer on tongue & mouth • Loosening of tooth after blow.

- Effective medicine for Skin disease, Itching on the folds of skin, Eczema, Ulcer on skin • Itching subsides within few minutes after application • High-grade pain reliever for all types of muscle pain & sprain (not fracture of bone), Pain & swelling due to blow • Relieves pain faster than other medicine • Partial benefit observed in tonsillitis, throat pain and sciatica • Good medicine for controlling diarrhea and vomiting (mix 30-40 drops MULTI-CARE and 5-6 caps SHAKTI-RAJ in a glass of water and drink frequently).

- Stomach problems are greatly reduced by brushing teeth with DANTA-RAJ toothpowder twice daily and applying 2-3 drops MULTI-CARE lotion on gum—gently rub by finger and swallow the medicine after application on gum.

- Medicine is having wide range of application • An essential medicine for family-stock • Excellent medicine for regular and emergency use.

AQUA-FRESH
HERBAL COSMETIC FOR SKIN & HAIR CARE

- An effective after-bath Herbal medicine especially for dry skin • Removes tiredness & brings freshness and comfort after bath (soothing & relaxing effect on nerves) • Acts as anti-bacterial and anti-fungal • Keeps skin healthy and retards aging effect of the skin • Roughness, cracks, itching, eczema, ulcers, boils, offensive odors, etc. are greatly reduced • An ideal lotion for herbal bath of small babies • An excellent and ideal cosmetic for ladies.

- Removes micro-particles of soap used during bath and the skin becomes smooth • Beauty of skin • Mix 2-3 full droppers in small quantity of water and pour on whole body after bath—medicine will keep the skin fresh and soft for both covered and un-covered area of the body • Local application on affected area • Good antiseptic after-shaving lotion.

- Effective medicine for preventing hair-fall due to dandruff or itching of scalp • Take AQUA-FRESH herbal bath daily and add green leaves (Chlorophyll) and coloured fruits in your diet to prevent hair-fall • Additionally take BIO-HERB 1 or 2, SUGAR-TABLET, BIO-TONE PLUS & BOOSTER and continue the medicines for few months.

- Essential lotion for all children, adults and especially ladies • It is to be noted that AQUA-FRESH is a dilute variety of MULTI-CARE lotion; hence it can also be used as an antiseptic and pain-relieving lotion • Thus AQUA-FRESH can be totally eliminated from Home-stock medicine.

HERBAL EYE-DROP
FOR TREATMENT OF EYE DISEASE

- Non-irritant type EYE-DROP for application in all types of eye disease—can be applied for indefinite period • Redness and irritation of eyes, Conjunctivitis, Glaucoma, Myopia, Optic atrophy, Vitreous opacity • Relieves stress for computer professionals • Protects eyes from excessive TV-watching, microwave radiation • Protects eyes from dust, retards development of cataract.

- For chronic eye disease, treatment with internal medicine as well as external medicine (eye-drop) proves to be most effective • Take BIO-TONE PLUS & BOOSTER at least for 10-15 days in a month for nerves and SHAKTI-RAJ liver tonic (must be taken for Glaucoma) regularly • Additionally take plenty of BIO-HERB to expel accumulated toxins from your body • For better control of bile take SUGAR-TABLET or LIV-TREAT daily • Brush your teeth by DANTA-RAJ toothpowder twice daily (to keep optic nerve healthy), apply MULTI-CARE lotion on your gum and swallow the medicine.

- Children can easily get rid of spectacles or improve their eyesight by taking BIO-TONE PLUS, BOOSTER & SHAKTI-RAJ medicines on long term basis (for detail of treatment Chapter-3 of the book is to be referred).

- Do not store the eye-drop for long—use fresh bottle for application • Remember the alternate arrangement—mix 10-15 drops MULTI-CARE or 3-4 droppers AQUA-FRESH lotion in a glass or cup of water and wash your eyes; you will get the same result of eye-drop • In case of urgency direct application of 1 or 2 drops MULTI-CARE or AQUA-FRESH on eyes is also recommended as a good alternative to eye-drop • Thus herbal eye-drop can be totally eliminated from Home-stock medicine.

FEVER-COLD & STOMACH-STOOL USEFUL MEDICINE FOR CHILDREN

FEVER-COLD: Liquid medicine for common cold, cough, running-nose, irritation of throat, viral fever, etc. • Itching sensation of skin, nerve-pain, muscle-pain • In case of bleeding from cuts and wounds, take medicine 5-6 times daily for 3-4 days and apply MULTI-CARE antiseptic lotion on the affected area—no infection or pus will be formed • Excellent medicine for children and babies for cold, cough & fever.

STOMACH-STOOL: High-grade liquid medicine for all types of stomach problems such as indigestion, acidity & gas, diarrhea, dysentery, pain in abdomen, bleeding of piles • Chronic dysentery for many years (for better result take SUGAR-TABLET or LIV-TREAT on regular basis instead of Stomach-Stool) • Good medicine for treatment of children and babies • Apply repeatedly till the problem subsides.

- Both medicines are complimentary to each other and cover wide range of problems • Favorite medicine of many people for application to their children because they need not think about symptoms—simply apply and get result.

- It must be remembered that BIO-TONE PLUS and BOOSTER must be applied instead of FEVER-COLD where fever is a result of complication due to tonsillitis, throat infection or unknown causes • Thus you can practically eliminate FEVER-COLD medicine from Home-stock.

SONALI
HERBAL ANTISEPTIC CREAM

- Powerful antiseptic, Anti-hemorrhagic, Anti-inflammatory, Anti-fungal Herbal cream • Stops bleeding immediately from cuts and wounds (in case of excessive bleeding, apply with cotton and bandage) • Heals cuts and wounds very rapidly • Burns from hot oil—no blister will appear • Bites from poisonous insects e.g. bees, wasps, ants, etc.—pain and inflammation will be subsided within few minutes • Itching of the skin, swelling, boils, dry eczema • Barber's itch • Muscle pain due to injury (not fracture or degeneration of bone—apply mild heat) • Headache from mental tension • Herbal cosmetic for ladies—excellent cream for cracks on feet or skin.

- An essential antiseptic cream for family—faithful friend of all housewives and children • Ideal cream for First-aid application—must keep this cream in your home-stock • It is the best medicine for bites from poisonous insect.

- This medicine is for external application only—do not apply on eyes or mouth.

COMMON KNOWLEDGE TO REMEMBER

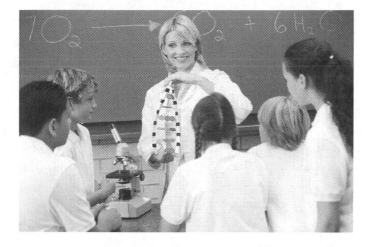

1) **SURGERY**: Where surgery is essentially required, undergo surgical treatment without hesitation. Remember, surgery is the oldest method of Ayurvedic Treatment originally developed by *Charak* and *Sushruta*. In doubtful cases, first apply the medicine—if it fails, undergo surgical treatment.

2) **EMERGENCY**: The cases need detail investigation and instrumental support—therefore, hospitalization is preferred. Additionally active and potent allopathic medicines may be required under guidance of specialist doctors. Emergency cases should not be treated with traditional systems of medicine.

3) **PREVENTIVE MEDICINE**: Use the preventive herbal and ayurvedic medicines lifelong to minimize the risk of "complicated" and "dreadful" diseases. Toxins accumulated in

your body must be expelled everyday. The role of herbal and ayurvedic medicine is to expel the toxins from body—thus ensures better health. Remember the old proverb—"Prevention is better than cure".

4) **DIET & EXERCISE**: Importance must be given to the "appropriate diet" and "exercise" for maintenance of health and also to achieve smooth and rapid cure of your disease. Take plenty of "Green Chlorophyll" and "Coloured Pigments" available in the Nature in the form of salad or 1-2 glasses fresh fruit juice or non-toxic coloured flowers in empty stomach. Remember these "pigments" are often called as "natural medicines" and are available in green leaves, coloured fruits and coloured non-toxic flowers. Reduce animal protein and fat intake; instead add more vegetables in your diet. Consult dietician for suitable diet. Do not overeat—take limited food and remain healthy. Try to do light exercise such as walking or jogging instead of doing vigorous exercise.

5) **DIETARY FIBER**: It is an essential item to increase longevity. Fiber also helps detoxification and removes the accumulated toxins from your body. Your diet should contain sufficient amount of dietary fiber. Additionally supplement the requirement of fiber by taking herbal and ayurvedic medicines.

6) **DETOXIFICATION**: It is the fundamental method of treatment, especially for the chronic or long-lasting diseases. Disease is caused mainly due to accumulation of toxins in your body—either from external source (from water pollution, food pollution, air pollution and microwave pollution) or from self-generated source (such as constipation, improper digestion or weakness of liver and kidney). One should therefore undergo detoxification on everyday basis to purify blood. Take plenty of water in empty stomach in the morning; add sufficient green and coloured vegetables and fruits in your diet. Take preventive herbal and ayurvedic

medicines lifelong for purification of blood—thus increasing immunity of your body.

7) **BASIC CARES**: Remember the basic way of maintaining your health → Mouth-care, Stomach-care, Detoxification, Skin-care and Eye-care. These five basic cares can prevent complex and dreadful diseases, even avoids hospitalization. Use of preventive herbal and ayurvedic medicines is an ideal solution. Give special importance on "Diet" and "Purification of Blood" which is a part of "Stomach-care" and "Detoxification".

8) **DOSE OF MEDICINE**: All our medicines are non-toxic, no side effect is caused and no dosage is directed. The word "Dose" is meaningless to us—medicines are analogous to food or nutrient. Therefore medicines can be taken at any time in any amount we like. Take medicine as per severity of disease. There is no restriction of type of diet—you can take sweet, sour, bitter foods along with the medicine.

9) **SPECIAL CONDITION**: In case of acute disease such as viral fever of unknown type, severe cold and cough, bronchitis, pneumonia, tonsillitis, severe type of vertigo, erratic pain on nerve, migraine, sciatica, arthritis, all types of infectious disease, menstrual pain, etc. take initially high doses of "Bio-Tone Plus" and "Booster" (say 2-4 doses each type daily) for 2-3 days till the crisis period is over—thereafter take normal dose along with other medicines.

10) HOME-STOCK MEDICINES: Because of limited number of medicines (only 9 numbers basic medicine) it will be convenient for you to keep some home-stock for your family use. Note that medicines are of multipurpose type and one can apply the same medicine in many types of diseases. Thus your child or aged parents can use the same medicine for maintenance of health as well as for treatment of common diseases at home. In other words application of medicine is user-friendly in all respect.

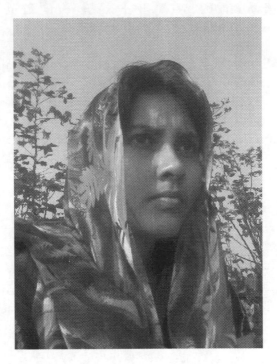

LIST OF PREVENTIVE MEDICINES FOR FAMILY-TREATMENT

ESSENTIAL MEDICINES FOR HOME-STOCK: BIO-TONE PLUS, BOOSTER, BIO-HERB NOS. 1 & 2, SHAKTI-RAJ, SUGAR-TABLET, MULTI-CARE, DANTA-RAJ & SONALI.

OPTIONAL MEDICINES FOR HOME-STOCK: LIV-TREAT, FEVER-COLD, STOMACH-STOOL, AQUA-FRESH & EYE-DROP.

NOTE: Medicines are not applicable for emergency, surgery or high-order genetic diseases.

LEARN FIVE CARES

FIVE "BASIC CARES" CAN PREVENT COMPLEX & DREADFUL DISEASES; AVOIDS HOSPITALIZATION AND SURGERY IN LIFE—"MOUTH-CARE", "STOMACH-CARE", "DETOXIFICATION", "SKIN-CARE" AND "EYE-CARE".

BRAIN TEASERS FOR STUDENTS OF SCIENCE AND NUTRITION

CATEGORY: EASY TYPE (10 QUESTIONS)

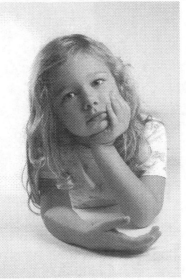

Q 1) Name at least three fundamental causes of disease. Justify your answer. Whether reduction of saliva has any role on disease?

Q 2) What are the sources of toxins? Whether you can avoid toxin in your body accumulated from "external source"?

Q 3) Micro-inflammation or irritation of body cells causes disease. True or false? Toxin causes micro-inflammation of cells. Justify.

Q 4) Name the most important process to eliminate toxin directly from body. How will you expel toxin on daily-basis?

Q 5) What are the "natural medicines" for human body? Name commonly available "natural medicines" in market.

Q 6) Name the sources of natural medicines. How will you add these medicines in daily-diet?

Q 7) Importance of Protein in diet reduces after 40 years age. Justify. Under what circumstances protein-based Nitrogen becomes harmful to your body?

Q 8) What is the normal pH of gastric juice? Which foods make gastric juice less acidic or in other words relatively alkaline?

Q 9) Intake of acidic food is one of the major causes of human disease. True or false? Why strong teeth indicate the healthy state of body? How will you prevent reduction of saliva of mouth?

Q 10) What is the difference between Chemical Energy and Bio-energy? Prepare a dietary chart considering more amount of Bio-energy.

CATEGORY: TOUGH TYPE (10 QUESTIONS)

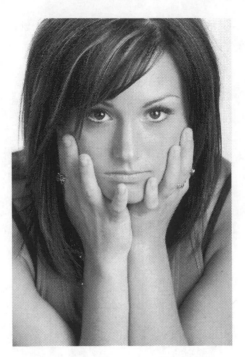

Q 1) List out the important causes of disease as per your judgment. Try to calculate the percentage (%) of its effect on causes of disease considering sum-total as 100%. Justify your calculation considering modern civilization and lifestyle of people. Will you consider psychological factor as one of the major causes of disease?

Q 2) What is bioflavonoid? List out the applications of bioflavonoid for treatment of disease and maintenance of health. What are the natural sources of bioflavonoid? What is the role of Chlorophyll in human life? What is pro-vitamin?

Q 3) Normal person requires about 2500 Kcal per day. Can you prepare a diet chart where he or she can maintain normal activity with about 1000 Kcal? Is it possible to remain healthy with a very low Calorie say 600 Kcal per day?

Q 4) Why less amount of Bio-energy is required compared to Chemical Energy for normal function of body? Find out the scientific outlook why Bio-energy is more efficient than Chemical Energy.

Q 5) Identify the foods which will make your diet more alkaline. What are the merits and demerits of alkaline food? What is the role of dietary fiber in maintenance of health? Under what conditions nitrogen of Protein proves to be more harmful than carbohydrates?

Q 6) Prepare a diet chart for a patient having Type-2 diabetes. Make diet charts for patients suffering from gastritis, arthritis and cardiovascular disease. Assume that the patients are not taking any herbal, homeopathic, ayurvedic or allopathic medicine.

Q 7) Compare between two major factors responsible for disease i) Genetic-factor and ii) Environmental factor. What is genome? List out some high-order gene related disease. How genes are responsible for cardiovascular disease and diabetes?

Q 8) Why susceptibility to become sick is directly related with genetic-factor or genetic-clock? One of the two persons is having life-expectancy 75 years and the other is having 120 years. In your opinion who will suffer more from complex disease and from which age?

Q 9) What is immunity system? How it takes part to prevent disease? What are the immunoglobulins? How antibody combats with antigen? What are the methods of elevating the immunity potential of your body? Try to establish relationship between "metabolic disorder" and "immunity potential" of body.

Q 10) How far genetic predisposition of disease can be controlled or reduced by natural medicines? How you can increase longevity and lead disease-free life?

HINT:

All above are general questions. Solve the questions without considering the methodology of treatment of disease. Note that there is no direct answer for "Tough" category questions and therefore, these are likely to have multiple answers. Apply your own logic, judgment and experience in life to find out the answers.

MISCELLANEOUS INFORMATION

FOR GENERAL COMPOSITION OF MEDICINES REFER
WEBSITE www.homemedicine.in

LEARN MORE ABOUT "BIOPATHY SYSTEM OF
MEDICINE" FROM OUR WEBSITE

CONTACT:
S. B. HEALTH GUIDE
Block-EB, Plot-64, 1848 Rajdanga Main Road
Kolkata-700107, India. Phone: +919433931994
e-mail: easymedicine12@gmail.com
biopathy1@gmail.com
Website: www.homemedicine.in

ALSO CONTACT US FOR "DIRECT" OR "POSTAL" OR
"E-TUITION" FOR PRELIMINARY KNOWLEDGE ON
VARIOUS SYSTEMS OF MEDICINES

REMEMBER, DISEASE MAY BE MANY BUT MEDICINES
ARE SAME

SELECT MEDICINE WITHOUT CONSULTATION
→ MEDICINES ARE PRACTICALLY SAME FOR
HOME-TREATMENT → JUST KEEP SOME HOME-STOCK
FOR FAMILY-TREATMENT

EASYMEDICINE BOOK IS A COMPLETE GUIDE FOR
HOME-TREATMENT AND MAINTENANCE OF HEALTH

AN EASY SOLUTION OF HOME-TREATMENT OR
FAMILY-TREATMENT

TAKE PREVENTIVE MEDICINE LIFELONG AND AVOID
SURGERY AND DREADFUL DISEASES IN LIFE

KEEP HOME-STOCK OF MEDICINES FOR MAINTENANCE
OF HEALTH OF YOUR FAMILY MEMBERS

FACILITY OF GETTING MEDICINE BY COURIER SERVICE
OR HOME-DELIVERY IS AVAILABLE FOR OUR PATIENTS

READ "EASYMEDICINE" BOOK TO LEARN THE SCIENCE
FOR HOME-TREATMENT

FREE-CONSULTANCY SERVICE FOR ALL:

BRIEFLY INDICATE YOUR PROBLEM AND MAIL US AT
FOLLOWING E-MAIL ID:

easymedicine12@gmail.com

OR

DIRECT CONTACT: +919433931994

• HERBAL • HOMEOPATHY • AYURVEDA • BIOPATHY •

HEALTH IS WEALTH

About The Author

He advocated amazing curative power of *natural medicines* i.e. green chlorophyll and coloured pigments naturally available in green leaves, fresh fruits, vegetables and nontoxic colored flowers. He considered the *natural medicines* as the purest form of bio-force or bio-energy for prevention of dreadful diseases. He also developed user-friendly home-medicine for family treatment.